Online Health Surfing

Online Health Surfing

Trends, methods and insights in Internet Health Information

Spencer D. Kroll M.D., Ph.D.

iUniversity Press
San Jose New York Lincoln Shanghai

Online Health Surfing
Trends, methods and insights in Internet Health Information
All Rights Reserved © 2000 by Spencer Kroll

iUniversity Press
an imprint of iUniverse.com, Inc.

For information address:
iUniverse.com, Inc.
5220 S 16th, Ste. 200
Lincoln, NE 68512
www.iuniverse.com

This text does not seek to endorse or encourage the use of any
particular web site or internet business. Similarly, this text is not
resposible for health care decisions or outcomes.

ISBN: 0-595-13340-1

Printed in the United States of America

To Nona.

Table of Contents

Foreword

As an Internet user, you may be overwhelmed with the amount of health related information that is available at your fingertips. The Internet has dramatically changed healthcare delivery by empowering the health care consumer to an unprecedented level. We are in a new era, in which we can take responsibility for, and control of, our wellness and illnesses. Online Health Surfing will provide you with comprehensive information regarding the options available for researching Internet based health information. There are now over 18,000 individual web sites offering health care information. The sheer volume of information—from alternative health treatments to doctors offering on-line treatments and advice is too overwhelming for the average individual to sort through. As a practicing physician, I confront patients' misunderstandings of web-based health information on daily basis. Most physicians are not computer-savvy and are also overwhelmed with the speed and volume of information that is disseminated on the Internet. After reading this book, you will feel comfortable turning to the web during an illness for health information. You will be able to integrate practical advice from experts regarding medical treatments into your health care and feel empowered to do so, by referencing information from quality sources when you discuss your health with your physician.

The reader will learn objective methods for evaluating the quality of online health information. He will learn methods for discriminating legitimate information from the large amount of "junk" that is readily available. The complex issues of medical privacy and security will be addressed and readers will learn new ways to manage their own health information on the Internet. Readers will learn how to find important information about their doctor or hospital that will arm them with sophisticated treatment decision abilities. Readers will also learn how to communicate the fruits of their research to their doctor without overwhelming the doctor or putting the doctor in a defensive position. Readers will learn how to seek out others with similar health concerns and how to collectively use this information to improve their health. After completing this book, the reader will gain insight into the limitations of web-based health information. Readers will have the confidence to locate credible information and useful products from trusted sources and integrate these findings into their healthcare.

One of the things that I strove for in writing this book was an avoidance of website reviews. There are many, many published books that give you up-to-date web site reviews. Additionally, several programs and search engines can direct you to health care web sites that have been "reviewed" and "rated". It is my intention to provide you with insight into the general trends that are occurring in online health research.

Preface

This book is designed for those people who feel comfortable using the web to gather information. You do not need any prior medical knowledge or other technical knowledge. People who are curious about how to discriminate the quality of on-line health information could read this book. People with legitimate medical concerns, whether they are related to an illness or strictly preventative could use this book as a source to enhance their experience when accessing on-line health information. Those who want to feel empowered regarding health care information and those who want to merge the latest technology with their daily lives should read this book.

Acknowledgements

I wish to thank my wife, Nona Balaban Kroll and my two children Ariel and Juliana, who put up with me. Thanks to Roxanne Bogucka, who edited most of the text, Kate Ewing, Jan Davidson and the rest of the people at NotHarvard.com. Also, I want to thank my father for buying me my first computer (a TRS-80!)—with 4 kilobytes of memory.

Introduction

Many consumers are moving away from traditional sources of health information, such as bookstores, libraries, and doctor's offices. They're finding new ways to gain insights into health and disease—online information. According to current estimates, about 18,000 web sites offer health care information. The vast majority of these sites are geared toward health care consumers. In the last year there's been a virtual explosion of information resources for patients. Clearly, we are witnessing a transformation of certain aspects of health and medical care.

Why are consumers turning to the Internet for more of their health information? The simple answer is, because it's there. More and more people use the Internet every day. But there are other, more complex reasons. Doctors have less time for each office visit, so patients get less time to discuss their concerns. Also, the business concerns that drive today's health care services leave many people looking for ways to participate in medical decisions. They see themselves as empowered health care consumers instead of as passive patients. Lastly, because a web-based health resource bypasses some of the more traditional providers of information, it streamlines the health care process.

The most significant outcome of this phenomenon is the emergence a breed of consumers who demand the most important, most up-to-date health information. These consumers choose Internet search engines over librarians, encyclopedias, and sometimes their own doctors. But Internet health information must be used with care. Not all health-related web sites are created equal.

I have been lucky to "grow" up in the Internet age. I started programming computers as an adolescent. I have witnessed the way that computers have edged their way into our everyday lives. In no way is this more true than in the delivery of information. Whether this information is stock market updates, travel information, consumer purchasing or medical information, we now have instant access to seemingly limitless amounts.

While it is by no means an absolute rule, medical problems tend to occur as we age. Many elderly people as well as baby boomers are now turning to the Internet for medical advice. Unfortunately, many of these people have little computer skills and are sometimes overwhelmed by technologic complexity. The loads of available information simply add to this sense of being overwhelmed.

I truly believe that all this information will improve a person's medical well being. Access to up-to-date treatments, discussions about differential diagnosis or simply resources for tracking disease prevention will enable people to have maintain a sophisticated involvement in their own health.

It is my hope that this book will provide you with the tools to improve your medical well-being.

Spencer Kroll M.D. Ph.D.
Washington, DC

Chapter 1.

Gateways to Online Health Information

According to Internet industry research, nearly 28 million people cruised the web for health-related products or services in 1999. About half of them purchased a health-related item. As the number of users grows, so do the number and kind of health information sites—an information overload that confuses and frustrates Internet users. A typical health-related search yields links to Internet portal health sites, consumer-and physician-based web sites, online pharmacies, disease-oriented web sites, and alternative medicine and nutrition web sites

Internet portals—gateways for searching the web—are the starting points for most net surfers. Many offer search engines and subject directories, as well as news headlines, weather forecasts, chat rooms, and shopping. In response to customer demand, portals like MSN.com, Excite, Go, Alta Vista, Lycos, and Yahoo! provide health information centers that offer search capabilities, breaking news, and disease-specific information. Visitors can search by disease or by particular health topics. Several offer advanced services to better meet patients' needs. Many search engine portals now provide breaking health news on a daily basis

Alta Vista, for example, has a "Health and Fitness" category. Clicking this category takes you to Intelihealth.com, a media company formed as a joint venture between Aetna U.S. Healthcare and Johns Hopkins University. Intelihealth.com offers search capabilities, articles, and daily health news, as well as resources such as a physician locator, a drug resource center, and a medical journal database. Other search engines lead you to individual practitioners and local treatment centers.

Consumer-oriented web sites are another realm of health-related information. Sites such as drkoop.com, WebMD, and DiscoveryHealth.com are usually well funded and nicely designed. Consumer-oriented sites typically provide searchable databases and forums moderated by doctors or other experts. You'll find a wealth of information about an illness or preventive care. They may also offer chat rooms and bulletin boards, which can be important aids for those who are often isolated by their conditions. These sites get their income through advertising sales. Businesses place banner ads on these sites because of their high "hit" rates—their large numbers of visitors. These ads can be targeted to specific consumers. The terms you enter in a search engine or where you surf determines what ads are delivered to you. Online pharmacies such as PlanetRx.com and Pharmacy.com are outlets for patients to both buy medicines and find information about them. Some of these well-designed sites will tell you about drug interactions, new drug formulations, and indications, as well as alternative therapies. These companies make their money through direct sales of their products. They can "undersell" local brick-and-mortar pharmacies by selling in high volume over the Internet.

There are many web sites devoted to nutritional products and alternative therapies. HealthShop.com and eNutrition provide nutrition information and often sell diets and vitamin therapies. Sites such as Acupuncture.com and Homeopathy Online promote alternative therapies, with associated products for sale. The Internet provides exposure and income for the companies and practitioners associated with these web sites. Further discussion of pharmacy web sites and nutritional/alternative therapy web sites is provided in a later chapter.

Finally, there are disease-oriented web sites for patients with cancer, heart disease, or just about any major medical ailment. These sites provide consumer-based advocacy information, resources for up-to-date treatments, and sometimes, alternative treatments. Because these sites are often set up to sell alternative therapies, they should be scrutinized very carefully. What looks like a consumer-advocacy web site may in fact be a site where an alternative therapy is promoted over conventional therapy. There are, however, sites published by organizations such as the American Cancer Society or the American Heart Association, that usually promote up-to-date information and offer consumers an objective picture.

How the Internet Is Changing Health Information

As fast as online health information has grown, the leaps and bounds of medical research have been even greater. At the same time that new discoveries in therapeutics, diagnostics, and preventive care have transformed medicine, the Internet has penetrated the lives of us all, making vast amounts of information available to the end user.

In an attempt to generate quality results, medical research has traditionally created a system of checks and balances. The academic industry requires that a medical discovery be tried, tested, and subjected to a rigorous course of debate before its final release. Peer-reviewed research, for example, allows new medical findings to be scrutinized, often by competitors, before it's released to the public.

In the past 20 years, however, media sources, among which the Internet must be counted, have competed to deliver medical information to consumers as quickly as possible. Every day you can read, listen to, or watch news about the latest medical breakthroughs.

These are often results presented at medical meetings or conferences and released before undergoing strict peer review, or even results published in non-peer reviewed journals. The media—be they print, TV, or radio—"hype" the news to generate interest or higher ratings.

Medical journals have further eroded their own credibility by releasing "pre-print" versions to TV and newspapers. Almost every day, we hear of an exciting new finding soon to be published in a major medical journal. This level of excitement boosts the circulation of the journal. It also subtly influences scientists and medical researchers to try to get their data published in these "well-read" and oft-quoted journals.

Becoming an Active Participant in Your Health Care

The number of health information web sites is growing at such a rapid rate because there is consumer demand for them. More and more people want to take active roles in their health care. Whether you want to supplement your care, examine it, or replace it, the Internet provides the resources to do so.

Many web sites present information clearly and simply, so that consumers with no prior medical knowledge can rapidly find what they need or want. When armed with the tools to separate quality information from junk, savvy consumers can be their own best health care advocates. Even if it means challenging your doctor or insurance company, with reliable online research, no one suffers. The bottom line is that your health wins.

If, however, you fall prey to snake oil or use valid information to "play doctor," Internet information can be a hazard. Though it is a phenomenal educational resource, the Internet has its share of false or misleading information and sellers masquerading as medical professionals. It's important to get your doctor's advice about online health information. It's just as important, obviously, for your doctor to stay current with online health resources—both for his or her own continuing education, and to guide you to credible and helpful sources.

Understanding the Interests of Presenters of Online Health Information

Most medical web sites present information in a seemingly qualified and sometimes scholarly manner. Discussion groups and medical questionnaires may be hosted by qualified physicians, who may be board-certified and are often listed as experts in their field. Just remember, a dot-com site is a commercial venture. Physicians who offer their services or lend their names to these sites do so for tangible rewards. In the high-flying world of e-business, this is usually money. This is not to say that there aren't suitable objective alternatives.

There are many publicly run web sites that offer rigorously scrutinized information. These tend to lack the slick appearances of commercial sites. On some publicly run sites the interface may be difficult to work with. Further, the information can sometimes be overwhelming. This also differs from commercial sites, which have a vested interest in delivering specific information to potential customers. A commercial site may be geared toward selling a product or leading you to another site. The motivating factors can be hard to identify.

Web sites that require you register as a user have the most to gain. Registration information is one of the hottest commodities in e-commerce. The information these sites get—whether it's your name, your interests, or simply your zip code—will be compiled and probably sold. Who wants to buy this stuff? Businesses that want to target their sales efforts and get the most bang for their buck. They may market their wares to just one zip code or only to people who like boating. Worse yet, once you're registered, most web sites can attach data about your health information, that is, what topics you searched on their site.

A reliable starting point for web surfing is the National Institutes of Health (NIH). It maintains a consumer information page that presents links to reliable sites. Medical organizations and consumer groups also usually present reliable medical sites.

How Sites "Consumerize" Information

When judging the value of health information, consider how it's presented. You may see health information labeled as a press flash or a medical update, or even as an email delivering up-to-date information directly to you. Remind yourself that these web sites and emails were designed to grab and hold your interest. Whether your interest leads to a sale or a click-through to a site where they want you to go, the site's owners probably have a vested interest in what you do next. Advertising isn't the only form of promotion to watch out for. The hype that's generated around some medical information can be misleading and very often deceptive. Almost all seemingly objective medical information on large commercial web sites is delivered for a commercial purpose.

Some of the consumer-oriented web sites deliver information packaged with links to other sites, further blurring the line between junk and legitimacy. Some web sites offer information that includes medical analyses from professionals and experts within a given field. These may or may not include endorsements. Regardless, a web page now exists with a physician's name and a therapy, cure, or treatment. The page can now be web-indexed under both the professional's name and the treatment, allowing search engines to find this page when the appropriate search terms are entered.

Finally, web sites often ask you to register before you can access their information. Registration generally includes, at the very least, a request for your email address. You may soon find yourself inundated with email. "Spam" emails may be directed to you because of search terms you used or where you surfed on a given site. These emails have much the same purpose as the sales circulars and store flyers you get in your mailbox—to get you to come to a particular place, in this case a web site, or to buy a specific item.

How to Identify Useful Health Information on the Web

Surf the web for health information with some predetermined rules. It will make for a safer, more accurate and more effective search. Here are a few rules to help you be a savvy surfer of health care information.

1) Don't play doctor. There's no substitute for a personal examination and a one-on-one discussion of your condition and health goals. Your doctor is the only person who knows your medical history and test results.

2) Retain your privacy. Your messages and searches could be read by millions of people. Think twice before offering highly specific health and medical advice to others or making negative statements about a physician or healthcare provider through a newsgroup or mailing list. You could be held liable for your comments. It may be best to share your personal experiences anonymously.

3) Don't act blindly. In many cases, you won't know who's behind the information you're reading. Scrutinize statistics and claims closely. Look for other reputable studies that offer the same or similar advice. Check out claims with your physician or a reputable source available on another site. Don't act until you've thoroughly checked out the information.

4) Get acquainted with large sites first. Search engines and large commercial sites can give you a general idea of what information is available. Many large sites are associated with reputable government agencies, universities, medical centers, or healthcare consortiums. Always check sites such as the NIH first. Much

of their information may be too complex for the medical layperson, but they can point you in the right direction.

5) Don't become addicted. In medical school, all students think they have every illness in the book. It's easy to become overwhelmed and think that a constellation of symptoms is a serious medical condition. Discuss your findings with your doctor. He or she spent many years getting a medical degree.

6) Develop a close relationship with your physician. An Internet search is no substitute for seeing your doctor. Your primary care physician can and should be able to guide you in your web searches.

7) Be skeptical. Be especially suspicious of people who make extraordinary claims or ask you to send money. If claims sound suspicious, request information on credentials and background.

8) Do some preliminary research. All kinds of people participate in discussion groups and support groups. Try to find out whether you're dealing with qualified professionals, other patients with similar problems, or just someone with something to sell.

9) Be careful. Be suspicious of people who refuse to give their real names and credentials on a web site or through a signature at the end of an email. Be wary of those who continually champion one treatment or course of action over another; or who seem to have a grudge against the medical community, healthcare system, or a specific company.

10) Know when to be specific. The best way to get an answer in a chat room or discussion group is to ask a highly specific question. (Just don't ask anyone to provide a diagnosis or recommendation on your condition.) The reverse may be true of a web site, however. Many web sites are deluged with visitors and have a huge backlog of questions to answer. A question that's

too specific may not be answered. A question that may apply to many consumers is likely to get answered sooner.

11) Be realistic. You won't find the cure for cancer or an instant solution to your healthcare problems on the Internet. What you will find are opportunities to conduct online searches for specific medical information, to track down experts on rare diseases, to get support from others with the same condition, to get information on clinical trials, to track late-breaking medical news, and to explore alternative therapies.

Chapter 2.

Searching for Medical Information

You'd think that an effective search strategy would consistently yield clear, concise results, but not all search engines are created equal. Different search engines index sites in different ways. Some search engines deliberately exclude certain sites—either because they contain misleading or false content or because the search engine host has an interest in keeping you away.

How do search engines work? When a web surfer enters a search term, the search engine uses any one of several algorithms (mathematical formulas) to search either its own pre-catalogued group of sites or the web as a whole. The most-used search engine, Yahoo.com, searches only for sites that are catalogued at Yahoo.

Altavista.com and Infoseek.com are two generalized engines that search the entire World Wide Web. These kinds of engines usually return a lot of hits on a search, but many of the results may not be relevant. Often, only a few of the search results actually match what the searcher was looking for. Engines like Google.com get around this problem by using an exact text match to find results, then looking at how many other sites link to those results in order the measure their relevance to the searcher.

How search engines search

How do search engines find individual web sites? The answer to this important question has implications for the entire structure of e-commerce. All web pages have an embedded code called a META tag.

This is usually a series of keywords that describe the site's content. These hidden terms are used to index sites and produce search results.

Meta tags are the hidden words that allow the entire World Wide Web to be indexed and catalogued. These terms are embedded in each web page that you view with your browser. META tags do for search engines what book indexes do for readers—they tell where to find information on a subject. Here are the META tags for the National Heart Lung and Blood Institute home page:

National Heart, Lung, and Blood Institute, NHLBI, home page, heart disease, cholesterol, high cholesterol

lung disease, asthma treatment, asthma, blood, cardiovascular disease, high blood pressure, pulmonary, pulmonary disease, hematologic disease, sickle cell, sleep, sleep problems, insomnia, sleep apnea

Web site creators can abuse the META tag by repeating the same word over and over. The more often a term appears in a META tag, the more likely it is that that site will be pulled up in a search on that word. Some people use terms in their META tags that have nothing to do with their sites, just to bring in viewers. This is a particularly severe problem in health care searches. Disreputable site creators often use incorrect, inaccurate, or misleading META tags. All you see, however, is that the site appears to match your search.

Some search engines that catalog sites rely upon web designers to submit their sites for entry into the catalog. This screens out some of the abuse. Many search engines, however, use a technology called a **spider** that crawls through the entire World Wide Web, cataloging individual sites. This automated process saves time and money for personnel to examine and scrutinize every web site in a catalog. Many health web sites use these types of search engines. These engines provide up-to-date information, but often return an overwhelming number of results.

Designing your search

There are two parts to a successful on-line search: A well-formed set of search terms and an accurate, reliable result. Most search engines allow you to use Boolean to focus your search: Most web searchers start their searches at large portals or search engines such as Yahoo.com or Lycos.com. The basic rules for entering search terms can be found by clicking on a site's help button. Typical searching rules are shown in the chart below.

Boolean Operators

You can enter a word or string of words as search terms. But most search engines also let you organize your search using Boolean logic. The term **Boolean** refers to a system of logical thought developed by English mathematician and computer pioneer, George Boole (1815–64). You use Boolean operators by combining your search terms with AND, OR, or NOT. Using Boolean operators with your search terms makes your search more specific.

Boolean operator	How it works	Example	Result
AND (sometimes "+") or just a space between words	Finds documents containing both words it joins	vitamins AND pregnancy	Sites containing both the words vitamins and pregnancy
OR	Finds documents containing either of the words it joins	vitamins OR pregnancy	Sites containing either word, vitamins or pregnancy
NOT (sometimes "-")	Finds documents containing the word preceding it and excludes documents containing the word that follows it	vitamins NOT pregnancy	Sites containing the word vitamins but excluding those also containing pregnancy

Other operators that work in many search engines include:

Boolean operator	How it works	Example	Result
, (comma)	Finds documents containing at least one of the words specified, ranks them using word-count approach, so documents with the most usages of the search terms get the highest rank	vitamins, pregnancy	Sites containing either vitamins or pregnancy; sorts results according to relevance
?	Represents any one character	?lood	Sites containing the character string lood preceded by one character, (e.g., blood, flood)
*	Represents one or more characters; cannot use * to specify the first letter of a word	heart*	Sites containing the character string heart(heartburn, heartache, etc.)
"" (double quotes)	Finds exact matches only	"gene"	Sites matching the word gene only (not genealogy, general, generate, etc.)

How to Improve Your Searches

Improve your search by following some basic rules. This will increase the power and accuracy of your search and deliver to you more comprehensive results.

BE SPECIFIC

Use specific terms such as **iron deficiency anemia** or **viral pneumonia,** rather than the broader terms **anemia** or **pneumonia**.

TRY ALTERNATE TERMS

Try alternate search terms for the same disease or condition (e.g., **alopecia** or **hair loss** or **baldness)**. Some of the medical web sites have online dictionaries you can use to find equivalent terms.

CHECK SPELLING

Search engines match exactly what you type. Think of alternate spellings such as **orthopedics** or **orthopaedics**, especially if you are looking for something from another country or language.

PUT PHRASES IN QUOTES

Use quotes for words that are part of a phrase (e.g., "systemic lupus erythematosis," or "aortic regurgitation"). This increases the power of the search and won't return sites that have each word individually scattered through them.

TYPE CAREFULLY

Check for typos. Make sure that you typed **heart**, not **hart**, or **diabetes**, not **dibetes**.

KEEP YOUR SEARCH NARROW

Use the minus sign (-) or NOT in front of a word you don't want to appear in the result. For example, **cancer NOT breast** will retrieve web sites on cancer, but none on breast cancer.

SKIP CAPITALIZATION

Search engines generally aren't case sensitive.

TRUNCATE TERMS

Truncation allows you to find variations of a word. Most sites use an asterisk as a truncation symbol. For example, **diab*** brings up results **diabetes**, **diabetic retinopathy**, **diabetic treatment**, and **diabetology**.

What Is There to Search?

Know the limitations of each search engine. Each one uses a different methodology to search the Internet or its own database. The same search terms on 2 different search engines can yield strikingly different results.

Search engines can be portals or internal search engines within a web site. A portal such as Yahoo catalogs web addresses throughout the world wide web. A search for a specific medical subject gives you web pages from all over the world—informational pages, drug company pages, advocacy group pages, alternative therapy pages, etc. Internal search engines of web sites such as drkoop.com only search within their own sites. Queries of internal engines tend to give more specific information, but information that may have been filtered (see Chapter 1).

A search for **colitis** in Drkoop.com gives you several informational pages, including a dictionary definition. It also leads to suggested drug and surgical treatments, articles on the proposed etiology of this condition, and links to related medical conditions. drkoop.com ranks these results in decreasing order of relevance. Links also include a page describing a brand new drug approved for colitis and actual pictures of the disease. Once you start following the links, you receive banner ads for online drugstores, online physician locator services, and online health insurance. Clicking through to their drug store sponsor, Healthemporium.com, leads you to a page where you can buy drugs for colitis.

Some engines search specific databases of medical literature instead of the world wide web. Online searches of the medical literature are perhaps one of the biggest advantages of the internet. As recently as five years ago, searching the National Library of Medicine's archives cost significant money per hour of research. Now it's all free to web surfers. Several sites have links to Grateful MED or MEDLINE. These sites allow you to do comprehensive searches of databases of published medical information.

Published scientific works are held to a higher level of scrutiny than most information published on web sites. There's a large difference in the quality of health journals. An article published in **The New England Journal of Medicine** may deserve more attention than one published in a thinly circulated journal such as the **Syrian Journal of Medicine**. This is not to say that the latter doesn't contain accurate articles. It's just that many journals, rather than relying on peer review, solicit scientists to write articles. In all journals, however, a review article—an analysis of a disease, condition, or surgery—should be interpreted as such. It's really a disguised editorial of the current state of the discussed issue. The author of a review article isn't subject to any external verification and can write what he or she wants.

How can you use all of these resources most effectively? Here's a sample scenario.

An Online Search Example

This is only an example. You can develop your own powerful search protocols by following a similar path.

You are a 45-year-old woman who has been told by your doctor that you have a small lump in your breast. The doctor suggests a fine needle aspiration/biopsy as soon as possible to rule out breast cancer.

Discussion: Clearly a cause for concern, you need information quickly in order to make a rational decision.

You might think www.breastcancer.com would be a reasonable place to start your search. This site, unfortunately, is a Chinese natural medicine site and offers a lot of misleading information.

www.yourdiseasehere.com

Unfortunately, you can't assume that a web site that goes by the name of a disease was created by an authority on the subject. Registration of site names has been haphazard and unregulated in the last few years. Anyone can apply for any commercial domain name that isn't already in use. Many "diseasename.com" sites exist to sell goods and services rather than to provide accurate health information.

The NIH website, NIH.gov, links you to the National Cancer Institutes and delivers a series of pages on breast cancer, including risk factors and early detection. From these pages, you can learn about the importance of your family history and how the location and size of the lump factor into your doctor's suggestions. All of this is helpful, but it represents consensus information published by NIH experts. It says nothing about alternative options and controversies in treatment.

The next place to stop is a large search engine. Using the search terms **breast** and **cancer** yields 397 websites. Many of these are international breast cancer treatment centers, clinical trial programs, and advocacy groups. Yahoo maintains its own health information area that gives a lot of good information, particularly on prognosis.

Refining your search to **breast** and **lump** yields only six web sites on Yahoo.com, including pages for mastectomy-related products, alternative therapies, and another Yahoo internal site for breast self-examination. Yahoo is one of the few web portals that will link you to other search engines if you need more results. Entering these terms into Infoseek, which searches the entire World Wide Web, returns more than 325,000 web sites. One of the top results is an excellent link to the Mayo Clinic's health information pages. These pages tend to be both informative and very readable.

Next, you might try one of the commercial medical websites. Again, using the search terms **breast** and **lump**, Discoveryhealth.com yielded many results from its internal pages as well as external links back to the National Cancer Institute. One of the discoveryhealth.com pages suggests important questions to ask your doctor. Refining your search at Healthcentral.com to **breast** and **lump** and **controversies** yields important information on alternative treatments and alternative screening regimens.

From the results of these searches, you can make some reasonably well-informed decisions about choice of care. You'll have appropriate questions for your doctor and insight into how he or she decided to recommend that you have a biopsy. Finally, if you have the misfortune to be diagnosed with breast cancer, you'll know where to turn for more information.

Ten Things to Know When Evaluating Medical Sites

All web sites are not created equally. Always be maintain a healthy amount of skepticism about each web site. Try to evaluate the reason why the information is presented to you on this site. Ask yourself these 10 questions when evaluating online information (adapted from the National Cancer Institute).

1) Who runs the website?

Any good health-related web site should make it easy for you to learn who is responsible for the site and its information. You shouldn't have to be a detective to get this information.

2) What is the purpose of the site?

This is related to who runs the site and who pays for it (see #8 below), and it should be stated clearly. Look for "About this site," or "Mission Statement," which are common titles for this type of information. If the site's purpose isn't to provide unbiased, accurate health information, be particularly careful about how you use what you're reading.

3) Where does the information come from?

Many health sites post information collected from other web sites or from offline sources. If the person or organization in charge of the site didn't create the information, the original source should be clearly labeled.

4) What is the basis of the information?

In addition to identifying who wrote the material you're reading, the evidence that material is based on should be provided. Medical facts and figures should have references (such as an article in a medical journal or the consensus of a meeting of experts reviewing research evidence). Opinions or advice should be clearly set apart from information that is based on research results.

5) How is the information selected?

Is there an editorial board? Do people with excellent medical qualifications review the material before it's posted? Information delivered to you should be reviewed by board-certified physicians or credentialed scientists. Leaders in their field usually have faculty appointments at medical schools or universities. Editorial boards should consist of several experts in a field.

6) How current is the information?

Web sites should be reviewed and updated on a regular basis. This information should be presented on each major page (e.g., "This page last updated on 7/9/99."). It is particularly important that medical information is current, and that its most recent update or review date is clearly posted. Even if the information has not changed, you want to know that the site's owners review it regularly to ensure that it's still valid.

7) How does the site choose links to other sites?

Web sites usually have a policy (often unstated) about how they establish links to other sites. Many medical sites take a conservative approach and don't link to any other sites. Some link to any site that asks, or pays, for a link.

8) Who pays for the site?

It costs money to run a web site. Although some sites are labors of love, most have an outside source of funds. Again, this should be clearly presented on the site. For example, a web address ending in .gov denotes a federal government-sponsored site. You should know how a site pays for its existence. Does it sell advertising? Is it sponsored by a drug company? The source of funding can affect the site's content, how that content is presented, and what the site's owners want to accomplish through the site.

9) What information does the site collect about you, and why?

Web sites routinely track the paths visitors take through their sites to determine what pages are being used. However, many health web sites ask for you to subscribe or become a member. In some cases this may be so that they can collect a user's fee (see #8) or select information that's relevant to your concerns. In all cases this will give the site personal information about you. Any credible health site that asks for this kind of information should tell you exactly what they will and will not do with it. Many commercial sites sell aggregate data about their users to other companies—information such as what percentage of their users are women with breast cancer, for example. In some cases they may collect and reuse information that is personally identifiable, such as your zip code, gender, and birth date. Read each site's privacy policy and don't sign up for anything that you don't understand.

10) How does the site manage interactions among visitors?

Sites should tell you how to contact its site owners with problems, feedback, and questions, and someone should respond to your messages in a timely fashion. If the site hosts chat rooms, it should tell visitors the terms of using this service. Is the discussion area moderated? If so, by whom, and why? It's always a good idea to spend time reading the discussion without joining in. Get comfortable with the environment before becoming a participant.

Chapter 3.

Online privacy and your health records

In **1984**, George Orwell described a central location where your thoughts or movements could be monitored. Little did he know that one day the Internet would make Big Brother a partial reality. Interested parties can find out where you surf and what you do on the web. They gather this information, analyze it, and create reports about you and your habits.

Perhaps the first big issue of the new millennium is Internet privacy. There are few rules and very advanced technology to track your health care surfing habits. Ad profiling analysis has tremendous implications for your online health research. In the race to build market shares and customer bases, many online companies ignore the consumer's rights to personal privacy. By the end of the 1990's, business valuations for online companies were measured by the number of customers their sites catered to—their audience reach. Today these valuations are driven by what these sites know about you. The number of personal profiles they build on individual customers enhances their marketing.

In some ways, advertising is the glue that holds the Internet together. One reason the Internet is readily and cheaply available is because advertisers can reach potential customers—us—in ways they could never before. Since the dawn of advertising, ad executives have devised ways to target their audience Whether it's a beer commercial during the Superbowl or a detergent poster at the supermarket checkout, ads are most effective when they're delivered at the right place and time. The Internet gives advertisers the chance to customize advertisements at an individual level. Advertisers gather information on where you go online to create a profile for you. The profile lets them deliver ads for products you're most likely to buy.

One way advertisers compile profiles is through the terms you enter into a search engine. Many search engines link what they know about you with your search terms. This information is then transmitted to online advertisers. It might happen instantly, so that ads are delivered depending upon your search request. More often, though, online advertisers have a complex and sophisticated profile that includes your current search, past searches, and surfing history.

Cookies, anyone?

A **cookie** is unique code for each web site. When you enter a new site, a new code enters the cookies folder in your computer. Online advertisers follow in your wake. They can check your cookies, instantly and invisibly, as you surf the 'net. A cookie may contain the name of the web site that issued it, where you visited on the site, passwords, and sometimes, even user names and credit card numbers.

The online advertisers argue that this service benefits you. It lets them deliver exactly the ads you want to see. Somebody has to pay for all this free Internet stuff. Free ads that are specifically selected for you may make it seem like you're receiving information more efficiently. All the extraneous ads are filtered out. But for online health care research, being able to surf the web in relative privacy and anonymity is an advantage.

Advertisers: Information Addicts

Typically, when you use a web site, you must register. This may be as simple as entering your email address. More often, though, it includes entering a lot of other demographic information. In 1999,

Georgetown University provided a study for the Federal Trade Commission with the following statistics on what items were requested for a wide range of sites.

It's obvious how your occupation or income could be used to profile you, but how do sites use your zip code or phone number? They can get information from the postal service and phone companies, which generate demographic information for advertising customers. What about the web site that asks for no information? How do they profile you? Every computer has an Internet Protocol (IP) address. This is a unique series of numbers that identifies your computer anywhere you go on the Internet. Sophisticated hit counters can track where you have been and important information about you simply based upon your IP address. Your IP address is readily accessible to all web sites whether you like it or not.

By now it's fairly clear that there are different views about giving out this information. Some people may benefit from receiving targeted ads by not having to listen to or look at things they don't want to. Others feel that requiring information when registering for a web site is a huge invasion of privacy and choose not to do so.

Pitfalls of Using Medical Terms in Searches

By now, you may have figured out that entering a term in a search engine affects which ads you get. The same applies to health-related searches of the Internet. Many search engines and medical web sites post privacy statements claiming that they won't sell your search habits or demographic information. What they don't tell you is that, while they don't sell information, their sponsors or advertising supporters have no such restrictions. Search engines and medical web sites can exist and offer their services for free because of the support of online advertisers.

I'm sure you've seen how entering a term in a search engine affects which ads you get. Both Infoseek and Lycos have the stated aim of creating a tracking system that would create highly detailed profiles of user search patterns. By matching the cookie ID with your profile, the web server can access your search history. Your patterns of research would be immediately apparent to anyone looking at your search profiles. If any form of identification were linked to these profiles it might prove a serious invasion of your privacy, not unlike having outsiders read the circulation records of library patrons.

Let's say an online profiling company has generated a sophisticated profile of your interests—they already know you like to visit sites about sailing or photography. Now you're submitting a search on heart disease, which will be added to your profile. Who has access to this information? At this point, we don't know. This controversial issue is being argued everyday and may eventually lead to governmental oversight. The problem is that restricting this information may weaken the entire Internet.

How can you play it safe? Later in this chapter, we'll discuss some tools and strategies you can use to ensure your privacy and sometimes your anonymity. Keeping your health information private is potentially more important than keeping your credit card numbers private. Insurance companies and pharmaceutical companies, for example, would love to know if you are surfing for information about heart disease. You could be a target for a heart medication ads. More ominously, your insurance company could decide to check into your health history before reinstating your medical coverage. Obviously health-related information, even in what seems like an innocent search, can have profound implications on your right to privacy.

Email Security and SPAM

Email has changed the world. In some ways, it has reestablished the art of writing. In other ways, it has increased demands on our time by requiring instant responses with little time for consideration. Emails are also a way for anonymous persons to send information to you. Much like the mailbox at home, your email can pile up with junk mail. In the Internet world, this junk mail is called SPAM.

Giving out your email address is a risky undertaking. It places you on advertisers' lists and guarantees that you will receive solicitations on almost a daily basis. Some of these may be important to you. They may contain updates on a topic you're interested in, offers for items in which you've expressed interest.

SPAMs for health care products are on the Federal Trade Commission's top 12 list of e-commerce scams. Use the same caution you would when judging print ads or commercials. Be skeptical of case histories of amazing cures or testimonials from "famous medical experts." Other red flags include products that are available from only one source or for a limited time, and phrases like "scientific breakthrough," "miraculous cure," "exclusive product," "secret formula," or "ancient ingredient."

Another troubling aspect of email is security. Most people's personal email isn't protected by the firewall of a network. Firewalls exist to shield security and privacy. Without a firewall, you can access your email from anywhere in the world. But so can hackers who have figured out your passwords. Some online advertisers track who you email and who you get email from. It's unclear whether advertisers have access to your email's contents. Most corporations and government agencies won't allow any information to be transmitted over online email. While some companies may allow sensitive information to be passed behind a firewall, most corporations and government agencies won't allow any information to be transmitted over online email.

You may not know that our email addresses are public domain information. Email harvesting technologies crawl the Internet every day, building and updating ever larger databases of email addresses. Furthermore, emails are commonly posted on bulletin boards at Internet health sites, allowing anyone to look at them.

Future Directions in Online Health Care Privacy

In a future chapter, we'll discuss online maintenance of and access to your personal health records. Many patients and their doctors already use systems to store and transmit private patient information, such as EKGs, x-rays, and charts, via the Internet. Clearly, there's s significant potential for loss of privacy. It's never wise to send private information about yourself, such as laboratory values or doctor's reports, unless you can verify the security of the server on which it is transmitted. To this end, the Federal Government has passed the Health Information Portability and Accountability Act (HIPAA). This law is intended to keep your health information from falling into the wrong hands, by ensuring that only the people who you authorize have access.

Since 1997, the Clinton administration has supported efforts by industry to police itself with respect to Internet privacy. In this climate, privacy seal programs have been developed to certify the compliance of web sites with privacy policies. But the public and legislators have become frustrated with the pace at which companies are joining and actually following such privacy programs. Indeed, to some it appears that privacy violations are becoming more widespread.

If industry privacy self-regulation can't get the job done, what's the next step? The answer appears to be twofold: legislation and market forces. A number of privacy bills have been introduced, including one that would prohibit companies from selling basic information such as names, addresses, and Social Security numbers of Web users without their consent. These protections would extend to cookies. Lawsuits have also been entered against companies that disclose personal information to advertisers without consent. These issues will heat up as we all continue to use web-based technologies for many aspects of our lives.

Media coverage of Internet security has been largely negative, and the discussions in the FTC hearings have likely fueled the anti-cookie fires. And cookies may already be becoming obsolete. Recent browsers give users the option to refuse cookies, and a growing number of add-ons allow one to disable them altogether. More than 60 companies, including Netscape and Microsoft, have agreed to a proposed system of collecting user information on a strictly voluntary basis. This would let you create your own profile, with your name, email address, hobbies and interests, and any other information that you want a web site to have.

Protecting Your Privacy on the Web

Protect your anonymity at all costs when surfing the Internet. Ensure your privacy with pseudonyms, private e-mail sites, cookie protection software, and a heightened sensitivity to potential loss of privacy. Several resources exist for surfing the World Wide Web anonymously. I also have a few suggestions for you.

1) When surfing for health information, create a pseudonym and a false email address. There are many web sites that provide free email. These include mail.com, xoom.com, yahoo.com and others. Create an email address that you use only for your health care searches. It may seem tedious, but it will protect your interests in the long run. Resist the temptation to forward the email from this address to your regular email. SPAMers can track you down this way.

2) Check out privacy web sites such as Anonymizer.com. This site offers software to surf the Web by blocking certain information that's normally passed freely between your computer and interested online sites.

3) Erase your cookies often. They're usually stored in your Internet preference folder in your browser. This is the folder online entities use to trace your Internet use. Also check out de-cookie-ing programs, such as WindowScrubber from Webroot.com.

4) Disregard all privacy statements on individual web sites. They are unregulated and often untrue. Sites also put online certificates on their web sites from supposed privacy experts and independent reviewers. According to the FTC, the companies that provide these endorsements are very often the same ones that want information about you.

5) Guard your password. It's the key to your account and your email. People who work for your service provider should never request your password. If they do, refuse the request and report the incident to your service provider immediately. Hackers have developed sophisticated programs that can guess your password based upon some simple characteristics that they feed in. It's fairly likely that they can pare down the potential list of passwords to your phone number, birth date, or spouse's name, so choose something less personal. Passwords with numerals and letters are harder to hack.

6) Be careful about revealing your Social Security, credit card number, or shipping address. Many web sites scramble or encrypt this kind of information to ensure the safety of your personal data. This technology is improving rapidly, but it isn't foolproof.

7) Don't put any information, particularly health information, in an email unless you are willing to have it posted on a bulletin board or read by others.

8) Never open an email or an attachment in an email unless you know who sent it. Unsuspecting email recipients may inadvertently infect their computers with viruses. Further, most SPAMers place a "return receipt requested" on their outgoing

email. Opening the email sends a signal back to the sender that you are interested.

9) Opt-out whenever possible. Companies often make opting-out difficult (in some cases, virtually impossible). If you have the option to be removed from a list, take it. Practically speaking, there's little you can do to protect data such as addresses, which are already a marketplace commodity.

10) Keep things in perspective. While it's wise to be cautious, it's also important not to lose perspective. After all, tracking customer behavior means that web sites can provide better service in response to our needs. We also need to remember that we live in a world where our phone calls can be tracked via Caller ID and our grocery purchases monitored via universal product codes and ATM cards. For now at least, it may be that cyberspace affords us far more privacy than we're used to having in the real world.

Chapter 4.

Managing Your Own Health Care on the Web

Imagine that you're in a car accident far from home. You're unconscious when you arrive at the nearest emergency room. The ER doctors stabilize your injuries but they haven't a clue about your medical history. They don't know what medicines you take regularly or any of your allergic reactions to drugs. This happens all too often. Most people don't keep a list of their medications, let alone carry one in their wallets.

The Internet could solve this problem by letting those ER doctors see a comprehensive report of your health history. This might include your medications, the illnesses you're being treated for, your wishes regarding life-sustaining treatments, and your religious preferences. Armed with this information, doctors can make educated decisions that may save your life.

There are now several commercially available web sites that let you maintain your health information online. MyHealthRecord.com, for example, lets users enter their health information and store it in what's described as a secure online environment. Subscribers can specify who has access to this information—any doctor, the person's primary care doctor, or a spouse. Parents can maintain school health records online information. HealthMinder.com allows users to enter personal health information; including medications and dosages, and links this information to related sites and relevant articles. HealthMinder.com and other sites can remind you of important dates for health prevention (e.g., your annual mammogram).

There are several commercially available programs that allow doctors to maintain medical charts online, or at least to create patient-encounter visits. These sites let doctors access your notes from any remote site—be it from the office computer or a Palm Pilot on the golf course. When you call with a question or an emergency, doctors can look up your information online. These programs are typically integrated into larger office management packages that include medical billing or prescription transfer capabilities. Most of these packages are expensive, so doctors have been reluctant to use them. One solution is the web site, Docnote.com, which is free to doctors because it's funded by online advertising.

Paper medical charts are cumbersome. They contain records of every encounter you've had with a doctor, plus correspondence on your behalf from other doctors. Doctor-generated online charts may provide some benefits. They free up office space, and can hold your x-rays, lab values, EKGs, and other information. In the future, this important information may be transferable among doctors, to expedite your care.

Your Privacy and the HIPAA

With all of this medical information flying around the Internet, you may well ask, "How private are my medical records right now?" At first glance, medical records appear to be one of the few truly confidential areas in our lives. Laws in many states, and the age-old tradition of doctor-patient privilege, make it difficult for others to gain access to your medical records. But the laws contain exemptions. And you often lose the right to confidentiality in return for insurance coverage.

People both in and outside of the health care industry share your medical information. The scope of this access is growing, as records are increasingly being placed online. Generally, your records are obtained when you agree to let others see them. You probably signed a waiver or consent form when you obtained medical care. This waiver allows the health care provider to release your medical information to insurance companies, government agencies, and others. Insurance companies require you to release your records before they will make a payment. Medical information may be shared between insurance companies. Government agencies may request your medical records to verify claims made through Medicare or Social Security. Employers can obtain medical information about their employees by asking employees to authorize disclosure of medical records.

In order to simplify health care delivery, the federal government has contributed to the rush to move medical records online by passing the Health Insurance Portability and Accountability Act of 1996 (HIPAA). The intent of this law is:

"To reduce the costs and administrative burdens of health care by making possible the standardized, electronic transmission of many administrative and financial transactions that are currently carried out manually on paper."

This Act is extremely worrisome to many in the medical field— and to the many groups that have championed patient privacy and the security of medical records. HIPAA allows access to a patient's medical records by any person or group even peripherally involved with the medical care and treatment of that patient. The list includes doctors, but also social workers, pharmacists, insurance representatives, hospital administrators, lawyers, and marketing firms. To top it off, this access doesn't require your consent.

Another Big Brother-like provision is that HIPAA allows access to medical records that are related to the patient. Someone might be able to justify looking at the medical records of your relatives, neighbors, or other patients being treated for the same ailment as yours. Ultimately, the government will probably restrict the use of our medical records. The rapidity of Internet expansion has led to a certain loss of privacy in this arena at present.

There are several agencies and groups that are committed to preserving your medical record privacy. Many of them maintain web sites, including The National Coalition for Patient Rights (nationalcpr.org) and the American Health Information Management Association (ahima.org).

Online Questionnaires

Many large medical web sites contain surveys, polls, and questionnaires. These include questions such as, "Do you believe in Vitamin C for heart disease prevention?" These sites post the poll results for consumer information. In other cases, questionnaires may take the form of complex treatment decision trees. These questionnaires ask you about such subjects as sun exposure, heart disease prevention, or cigarette smoking cessation. Unfortunately, these questionnaires often lead users to sunscreen ads or nicotine patches. You get to compare your answers with others who took the questionnaire. Because of the vested interests of advertisers, though, many quizzes contain misinformation.

WebMD.com, one of the most popular medical web sites, has a 45-question general health questionnaire. You are asked questions about all aspects of your life from alcohol and seatbelt usage to your blood pressure and cholesterol levels. Your results are used to create a health risk profile for various diseases and a life expectancy forecast. Pfizer.com is an example of an interactive site that allows you to both manage your health information as noted above, and to save clippings of important articles and related research. This is bundled with online treatment decision tools (see next page), and an online health library.

Medical questionnaires exist as a learning tool—like any quiz, you may learn about your own misunderstandings or misconceptions.

Many websites use questionnaires to help you build on on-line profile, thereby directing you to appropriate resources. In some cases, these medical questionnaires are designed to guide you to certain information that may be in someone else's interest. As we will see, powerful treatment decision tools can also be used in this way.

Treatment Decision Tools

Treatment decision tools are some of the most helpful aspects of online health care. Many medical web sites provide interactive pages and forms that allow you to track the progress of your condition. Most sites contain a disclaimer such as:

Nothing contained in the results we present, based on your answers, is intended to serve as medical advice, diagnosis, or treatment. We do not directly or indirectly practice medicine, nor do we dispense medical services as part of this offering. Always seek the advice of your physician or other qualified healthcare provider before starting any new treatment, likewise with any questions you may have regarding a medical condition.

Many of the medical web sites that include these tools point to resources to improve your care. Intelihealth.com provides a sophisticated diabetes-tracking tool that gives you information on health screening intervals, necessary medication, and diaries for blood sugar monitoring. These tools work with you to promote proper management of your illness or answer your questions. Again, these may link you to banner ads related to your condition. Additional tools exist for conditions such as heart disease, HIV, and asthma. There are also treatment decision tools for preventive medicine decisions such as pregnancy management and weight management. These programs often lead you to support organizations and clinical trials. Please note, however that the information that you enter in these management tools can be used to profile you.

Some web sites have set up decision-making programs in the form of a laboratory. MyHealth.com has a section called the Allergy Learning Laboratory. Users can check their allergy symptoms and compare them to those of other users. Users can also keep logs of asthma/allergy symptoms, as well as objective measures such as peak airflow rates. Other sites contain free, downloadable treatment decision tools. Mayohealth.org has a blood pressure tracking program. While it doesn't actually take your blood pressure, it does let you keep a log that may help your doctor treat you.

Currently, there aren't any web sites that offer objective clinical information beyond what you type or submit. In a later chapter, we'll discuss doctors practicing online. An online doctor may offer you advice. A treatment decision program may arm you with a sophisticated analysis of your data. But so far, the Internet has not substituted for the actual examination of the patient—whether it's listening to a patient's heart or taking a chest x-ray. This form of remote medical practice may ultimately occur. One day your doctor may be able to make a house call over the computer.

Another health care information resource is MedicineNet.com. At this web site, there are listings and discussions of thousands of different lab tests. This site is indexed by test name and by disease. Further, patient questions about individual tests are posted on the site. This is one of the best resources for learning about a specific test, why your doctor ordered it, and what the results might mean.

Directed Email and SPAM

One of the fastest growing entities on the World Wide Web is directed email. Email is really a directed advertisement. By registering at a particular web site, you may have to give your email address. Once you do this, you're entered onto the web site's mailing list. You may be asked whether you'd like to sign up for medically related emails.

In some cases, however, directed emails alert consumers to important product updates or treatment information. You have to take the ads with the potentially important information. It is important, however, to check the source of these emails. A general guideline is to stay away from emails from advertisers. Mail that's not from a site where you're a registered user may be unreliable.

Email can also take the form of direct unsolicited promotions. You may have already received email from a source you can't identify. This is known as SPAM—a commercial email, often sent in bulk, and without consumers' prior request or consent. The Federal Trade Commission has published several reports on the growth of SPAM on the Internet, specifically in relation to health care. They conclude that well-known manufacturers and sellers of goods and services seldom send SPAM. Therefore, knowing the source of an email is the only really good discriminator. Email has been exploited by thousands of online hucksters as an innovative way to reach millions of consumers. SPAMs are more likely to contain false information about the sender, misleading subject lines, and extravagant performance claims about goods and services.

Chapter 5.

The Web and Doctor-Patient Communication

How to Approach Your Doctor with Internet Research

Patients are increasingly searching for and finding sophisticated health information from medical journals and medical web sites. This is a natural extension of all the health information now available. Doctors use this readily available information too, to update their knowledge and to search out alternative healthcare information.

Doctors are inundated with medical information. Whether promotional materials or patient's research, doctors sift through mountains of information, separating the good from the bad. No doctor likes being challenged on his or her decisions or knowledge—but the Internet provides a means of gathering information that your doctor may not be aware of. Additionally, you may seek Internet health information because of:

1) frustration about the amount of time the doctor spends with you

2) frustration about failed treatments

3) lack of trust in your doctor or health care system

4) a desire for anonymity, or feelings of embarrassment about a topic

Your Doctor as Guide

One doctor tells his patients that, "The Net is to peer-reviewed journals what the Wild West was to conservative old Philadelphia:

It's a place where the best and worst in information co-exist, and it isn't always easy to tell them apart." Doctors worry that patients may use spurious information to demand changes in their treatment plans. Doctors fear that the increasingly limited time that they can devote to patient care will be taken up answering patients' questions.

Many doctors are now steering patients to particular sites that they have previously evaluated. You should be able to gauge your doctor's willingness to discuss medical information from the Internet based on a few observations. Your doctor:

1) should accept your desire to supplement your medical care with online research, and should respect your wishes for autonomy and honor your initiative.

2) may inform you that while you may find information about a specific disease on the Internet, he or she has the training to analyze the data, using time-tested scientific criteria. He or she should be willing to use this expertise.

3) may react in a positive manner about information from the Internet but warn you that its quality and reliability are unknown.

4) may request that you send emails, as time constraints don't permit him or her to read pages of information during office visits.

5) should have a strategy for dealing with Internet information from patients.

6) should accept that you may possess valid information that he or she is unaware of.

7) should always be able to say, "I don't know, but I'm prepared to do the research and talk about it at a future time."

In my practice, I have developed a web site which links patients to medical information I have previously scrutinized. When patients come to me with their research, I steer them to my site and other credible sites for additional information. This saves me time and gives the patient a lot of quality information. Patients seem to like this pre-selection process. It seems clear that in the future, patients may choose their doctors based on both their responsiveness to Internet-based information and to their familiarity with Internet-based resources. Your doctor-patient relationship may already include discussions of online medical resources. According to a study by the Health On The Internet Foundation, 58% of patients say they discuss drug information they find on the Internet with their care providers.

How to Discuss Internet Findings with Your Doctor

Many doctors give patients evaluative devices to analyze the quality of the health care information. Doing a little homework may make your doctor more likely to discuss your findings with you. Among the tools available to you is the "IQ Tool" available at hitiweb.mitretek.org. This tool asks 21 questions in yes/no format, including questions about the author's credentials and the site's sponsors. The results are then tabulated and formatted into a report. Some doctors will only evaluate Internet health information if it is accompanied by such a report. Another tool is called DISCERN, available at discern.org.uk. This is a 16-question survey that helps users rate the reliability of sites. Your doctor will be much more inclined to discuss your findings if they are accompanied by such an analysis. Finally, there's an excellent discussion on reading medical articles at cmh.edu/stats/journal.htm.

I devised the following template to use when discussing Internet research with your doctor, based on health research my patients bring in.

Name of article or web site			
Is the author identified?	Yes	No	
Are the author's credentials identified?	Yes	No	
Is this a promotional site for a product or service?	Yes	No	Unknown
Are sources and references identified?	Yes	No	
Are the author's credentials or experiences relevant to the subject?	Yes	No	Unknown
Can you identify a sponsor for this page?	Yes	No	
Are financial biases or conflicts explained?	Ye	No	
Does the sponsor have any control over the content of the site?	Yes	No	Unknown
Is the information current?	Yes	No	Unknown
If you input information or submit queries in this web site, is a statement provided that explains whether or not this information is confidential and secure?	Yes	No	

When Online Sources Are More Informative Than Your Doctor

Your doctor should also be willing to discuss your Internet findings to some extent. Here are some warning signs that may indicate that a doctor's unwillingness to discuss your information.

1) dismissive or paternalistic attitude about your findings

2) derogatory remarks about others' comments on the Internet

3) outright refusal to discuss or view your Internet material

5) one-upping you with his or her own research

6) reaching patient confidentiality rules by defensively refer-
ring to other patients' problems or willingness to break
your own confidentiality to prove that he or she is right

Many doctors are overwhelmed by the amount of information
that they receive on a daily basis. Medicine is a life-long learning
process. A physician spends four years in medical school, but is
required to participate in continuing education every year and, in
many cases, periodic re-certification. Doctors who aren't willing to
integrate the latest medical information into their practices are not
worth seeing. A doctor may have tremendous experience or be willing to spend seemingly unlimited time with you. But if a doctor
agrees to treat you in any way, he or she is obligated to use current
knowledge for medical decision-making.

Doctors who are unwilling to use the Internet as part of their
practice are fighting an uphill battle. Whether it's simply integrating web-based information into their current knowledge or
adopting Internet technology for their everyday practice, doctors
should be willing to meet reasonable needs and requests. Studies
show that patients may be willing to change doctors at the click of
a mouse to get what they want. Most consumers expect their
physicians to be Internet-literate. You may have trouble assessing
your physician's clinical abilities, but you can determine if your
physician is well informed.

No doctor can have current information on every aspect of medicine. A doctor should, however, be up-to-date on the problems and
diseases he or she deals with most often, and should know the
advantages and pitfalls of alternative therapies. While doctors may
not have time to research esoteric information, they should extensively search the Internet for information about the 10 diagnoses
they encounter most.

Doctors, Patients, and Email

Whether your doctor embraces the Internet or resists it, one of the resources he or she is likely to use is email. Many doctors and patients happily use email for such tasks such as appointments, managed care referrals, and prescription refills.

In my practice, I use email to notify patients when test results are available, either with an indication that they were normal or an instruction to call me. We give patients a form that contains their email address and a consent release that allows us to communicate with them via email. Most patients are more than willing to use this service. In some cases, email communications allow us to skip routine follow-up appointments. Patients can print out an email and study it at their leisure, rather than in a hurried, information-packed phone call with their doctor.

Have you ever forgotten to ask important questions while you were in the doctor's office, or felt uncomfortable asking about something face-to-face? Email lets some people express themselves more effectively. Travelling patients can get in touch with their doctors while away from home.

A 1999 survey of 10,000 physicians by Healtheon found that 33% had used email at some point to communicate with patients, a 200% jump over the year before. Many doctors, however remain wary of email. They're reluctant to give out their email addresses for fear that they will be inundated. Patient emails could become a burden, requiring additional hours of work for no pay. I think it's important for doctors and patients to set the ground rules for email from the outset. Among the rules which I feel are necessary:

   1) Establish a policy for forbidden and private subjects. It's still unclear who has access to all the email flying around the Web. Be aware that you employer may have access to email you receive at a work address.

2) Set a reasonable turnaround time for response, based upon the nature of the problem.

3) Do not use email in emergency situations.

4) Be concise in your email communication. Describe your symptoms clearly. Almost all doctors will tell you that the patient's history is far more important than the physical exam in narrowing the differential diagnosis.

5) Keep copies of all email.

6) Don't cut-and-paste articles into emails. Only links to sites should be provided, so that the doctor can ascertain the quality of the information. You could, however, save your doctor some time by doing some of your own evaluation (see below).

Another exciting use for email is monitoring patients who either can't get to my office or don't need to come in. Applications are being developed that use email to communicate with homebound or disabled patients. Similarly, email could be used instead of an office visit for a patient who has a slight, often normal, change in symptoms or conditions.

The virtual housecall may become a reality using the growing convenience of the Internet and email. While the key to any technology is ease of use, patients must realize that this technology is a supplement to office visits and not a replacement.

I believe that doctors will soon realize that email can dramatically reduce the labor-intensive and often error-prone practice of phone tag, can speed routine transactions like prescription refills and delivery of lab results, and can create a record of consultations between clinic visits. Because email is a self-documenting process, it may be easier for doctors to bill insurers for online treatment advice. Email may have the most potential in capitated situations, where communication and timely intervention may prevent an expensive office visit or hospitalization.

That stated, there is a large medico-legal issue regarding email communication. Is advice given on by email binding? Does it constitute a situation where a physician can be held liable for misinformation or poor advice? What about interstate and international issues of medical treatment? Can a physician dispense advice in a state or country where he is not licensed? Or is a physician responsible for communicating with a patient he or she has never met face-to-face? There are no laws currently on the books for these important issues.

I believe that your doctor will soon realize that email can dramatically reduce established office practices such as the labor-intensive and often error-prone practice of phone tag. It could also potentially speed routine transactions like prescription refills and delivery of your lab results. Communication by e-mail followed by timely intervention may sometimes prevent an unnecessary office visit or hospitalization.

That stated, there is a large medico-legal issue regarding email communication. Is advice given by email binding? Does it constitute a situation where a physician can be held liable for misinformation or poor advice? What about interstate and international issues of medical treatment? Can a physician dispense advice in a state or country where he is not licensed? Or is a physician responsible for communicating with a patient he or she has never met face-to-face? There are no laws currently on the books for these important issues.

Most doctors chose their profession because they wanted to help people. One thing that every doctor appreciates is a grateful patient. The Internet also promises to facilitate this process. Pfizer.com has a tool for you to send a thank you note to your doctor. Additionally, tips on writing to your doctor are available at Writeexpress.com.

How to Involve Your Doctor in Online Research and Care

More and more consumers are looking for physicians who offer electronic services, such as access to blood test results. There's a growing sense that medical information should be as easily and readily accessible as financial information. Whether doctors will universally adopt such services is unknown. There is, however, huge growth in the development of applications for doctor-patient communication.

You can encourage your physician to use the vast resources of the Internet, by steering him or her to web sites that are geared to physicians. For example, your doctor could save vast amounts of time by subscribing to email updates from physician web sites such as Medscape.com, the Doctor's Guide to the Internet (pslgroup.com/DOCGUIDE.HTM) or Pharminfo.com.

When any new technology affects a long-standing institution such as the doctor-patient relationship, there are pluses and minuses. One advantage of the Internet is that it may reduce the number of calls a doctor gets because patients can find answers to basic questions themselves. While a doctor may not be able to find the magazine article or see the TV show a patient watched, the Web site the patient visited is easily accessible. This provides an opportunity for dialogue.

One danger of the Internet is that virtual contact will become a substitute office visit for some patients. Ready access to online health information may cause the uninsured to forego proper medical care. Although one would think that the uninsured would have less access to computers and the Internet, research by the American Medical Association indicates that they use online health information at a higher rate than those with health insurance

Traditional, face-to-face doctor-patient interactions may be replaced by other means of communication. In some ways, there will be a loss of intimacy with your doctor. In other ways, however, it will enhance the quality of your interaction by allowing your doctor to devote more time to you. The Internet is changing not only how doctors and patients obtain health care information, but also how they communicate with each other. The Internet can empower patients. If patients use the Internet and have more input into their health care, they will also have more responsibility in carrying out a treatment plan.

Chapter 6.

Searching for Doctors and Hospitals Online

Online information about a physician, hospital, or medical service can be divided into advertisements and evaluations. The growing penetration of the Internet into our lives and the ease of Internet advertising have led many doctors and hospitals to create their own web sites. These sites are promoted through registration with search engines, banner ads, and referrals from other web sites. The Internet also provides a means for evaluating physicians, including their disciplinary records, credentials, and patient satisfaction data. Consumers can compare treatment options and results within a geographic area by comparing hospitals. This allows users to make more educated decisions about where to seek care.

Doctors haven't always advertised. Traditionally, the medical community has looked upon advertising as unprofessional behavior. In the past, doctors might simply have an entry in the phone book. Referrals were made by word of mouth. Obviously, doctors are now selling their services directly. And they aren't the only health care providers to use more aggressive advertising. The airways and print media are jammed with direct-to-consumer ads for prescription pharmaceuticals. Furthermore, hospitals and insurance plans market their services.

Let your mouse do the walking

Managed care and the growing sophistication of consumers mean that more patients than ever search for doctors or health resources. The Internet is an excellent tool to locate physicians, medical services, and hospitals. Many health care providers have responded by creating their own web sites, links, and online tools for consumers, to attract more business.

Web site production is relatively inexpensive, so many doctors, even in solo practice, are eager to create an online presence. Many doctors now have modest web sites, with their name, address, office hours, and hospital affiliations. These sites might also include their email address and credentials. Research by the American Medical Association suggests the creation of a web site does not significantly contribute to the growth of a physician's practice.

Other doctors have leapt into cyberspace by creating web sites with informational links. I refer my patients to my web site, DrKroll.com, for further information on such topics as hypertension and diabetes. The site contains links to valuable resources at the National Institutes of Health and Georgetown University Medical Center. Other doctors' web sites provide valuable patient treatment decision tools, similar to those on the larger medical web sites. The Schering/Key Pharmaceutical Company will create web sites for doctors for free. The site itself contains no advertising from the company, but has links to other sites that do. According to the United States Inspector General, placing drug company ads directly on physician web sites is illegal.

Both doctors and consumers should know that web sites may create huge liability issues. Advertising claims in any form, whether written word or computer-transmitted text, are legally binding. The Internet is governed by the same ethical and legal rules that apply to routine medical practice. Doctors, for instance, are not allowed to offer online counseling to patients who live in states outside of those in which they are licensed. We will discuss physicians practicing over the Internet in another chapter

It's clear that the number of doctor's web sites will only continue to grow. The American Medical Association estimates that only a few thousand of its 650,000 physicians have their own website. Another study by Healtheon suggests that 30% of physicians have a website. To this point, these web sites have been completely unregulated in terms of their content and the scope of their use. Physicians are already restricted from self-referral. For example, a doctor may not refer a patient for a MRI if he or she owns an interest in the MRI facility. Similarly, there needs to be some form of oversight to determine what doctors can do with their individual web sites.

As more doctors consult with web designers, physicians' sites will increasingly contain slick design elements and easier-to-use interfaces. As web site design becomes more sophisticated and more doctors create web presences, consumers will need more tools to discriminate doctors' quality from the quality of their web sites.

Finding a Doctor Online

When your employer changes health plans or the doctor you've seen for 25 years drops off your insurance list, where do you turn? Your provider directory may provide little more than a doctor's specialty, address, and phone number. You may wind up choosing a doctor based on proximity. It's a challenge to differentiate one provider from the next and to find the one who can best meet your needs.

One answer is to use one of the many doctor-locator web sites. Most doctor-locator web sites contain disclaimers based upon referral. One site, Doctordirectory.com, offers point-and-click access to a listing of doctors' names, specialties, addresses, and phone numbers, as well as maps to offices, board certifications, medical schools attended, residencies, fellowships, secondary specialties, office hours, languages spoken, affiliated hospitals, and health plans accepted. Almost every practicing physician in the United States is listed.

Insurance company web sites also offer these services, allowing you to select a physician who is on their plan. A potential problem, however, is that health plan affiliations can be outdated as physicians initiate or terminate contracts. Remember that many sites will deliver targeted banner ads based on your physician search. A request for a gastroenterologist may mark you for an ad for diarrhea medication.

To locate a board-certified physician without receiving banner ads, try the American Board of Medical Specialties at ABMS.org. A doctor's board certification status is important. It provides you with assurance that the physician has successfully completed an approved educational program. Board certification includes an examination process designed to assess the knowledge, experience, and skills needed to provide quality medical care in a particular specialty.

Another aid to your doctor selection is seeing which health plans a doctor accepts. Many doctors are leaving certain health plans that they feel don't adequately reimburse them. Some doctors don't accept any form of insurance at all. Physicians whose reputations will attract patients to go beyond their covered providers have led the exodus from health plans. Beware of physicians who accept many different health plans. Similarly, beware of staff-type affiliations, where doctors may be restricted to only one health plan. Staff-model health plans tend to attract lower quality doctors. These health plans may also restrict the services their doctors can provide.

Doctors who use many health plans are more likely to be overbooked. In addition, these doctors are usually looking to grow the size of their practice. Doctors who work in staff model health plans are severely restricted by their health plan contracts to provide you with thorough comprehensive care.

A physician's license status is another factor patients should consider. Doctors are licensed by state. Using the Internet means that doctors could potentially offer advice and practice outside of their jurisdiction, which is illegal. The enforcement of interstate practice law has not caught up with the growth of Internet physician practice.

Consumer Ratings and Disciplinary Records Online

Another potential use for the Internet is for rating and evaluating physicians. One site, Healthgrades.com, helps you find a physician and shows you patient satisfaction feedback. This is somewhat subjective information, but it may be valuable to you. Right now, most doctors on the site have no evaluations, but this will probably change as more people go online. Physician evaluations by other physicians also have pitfalls. Many local magazines have lists of best doctors that are available online. The criterion for selection is often a poll of local physicians. This might be a popularity contest, rather than an objective evaluation. It may reflect how easily one physician works with another, rather than the actual quality of that physician's care.

The Internet is a useful resource for tracking the practice history of your doctor. Healthgrades.com provides physician disciplinary records. This information can also be obtained from the web sites of individual state medical boards. A physician who's had his or her license suspended or revoked has in some way abused the privilege to treat patients, resulting in this action. Possible offenses include incompetence, negligence, substance abuse, improperly prescribing drugs, fraud, improper sexual conduct with a patient, and criminal convictions. It's important to note that there may be a time lag between when a doctor is disciplined and when that information is reported. Here are some important terms to look for:

Probation: This is a period during which the physician is monitored while continuing to practice. Probation may be for a specified duration (often measured in years) or it may be permanent. This status is often accompanied by additional terms that place limits on the physician's practice. A physician who is under probation is also usually subject to continued monitoring by the state board.

Suspension: This is usually when the physician's license has been revoked for a limited period, during which time he or she is unable to practice medicine.

Revocation: This action is usually permanent. However, revocation does not always preclude physicians from practicing in other states in which they are licensed.

Surrender of License: Often, to avoid confrontations with the medical board or prolonged legal battles, a physician will voluntarily surrender his or her license to practice medicine in a given state.

The Internet does not allow physicians to hide their past problems. Consumers can find exhaustive information on license suspension and revocation as well as information on other disciplinary action.

Hospital Searches

Ratings that compare hospital performance are an important resource for health care consumers. Some web sites present this information to you so that you may compare hospital services. This can be valuable, for example, when considering where to have surgery. These measures do not translate to physician care only. They may include nursing care, hospital cleanliness, drug availability, and tertiary services such as x-ray facilities, respiratory care, and physical therapy.

An additional online tool to rate hospitals is the Joint Commission on Accreditation of Healthcare Organizations site (JCAHO.org). This organization is the nationwide authority that surveys hospitals. The JCAHO decides whether a hospital keeps or loses accreditation, based on certain health and safety requirements. Although accreditation is voluntary, most hospitals go through the process. If the hospital you are considering is not accredited, it's important to know why. For quality control, hospitals are required to report objective measures of health care. These are standardized measures, such as mortality for a particular operation or outcome from a specific therapy.

One of the major uses for the Internet is advertisement. Whether it is for products or services. Many doctors and hospitals have jumped on the bandwagon, rushing to form a web presence. As we will see in the next chapter, many other forms of health care are also using the Internet to get services to consumers.

Chapter 7.

Alternative Therapies, Discussion Groups, Patient Advocacy and Clinical Trials

Alternative Therapies

Like weeds in your garden, alternative therapy web sites continue to pop up on the Internet. The definition of a weed, however, is a plant that you simply don't like: One person's weed may be another's treasure. As a practicing allopathic (conventional) medical doctor, I don't generally espouse alternative therapies, but there are exceptions. I'm not going to address the merits of any individual alternative therapies. I will, however, give you some direction on evaluating these sites.

The Internet provides resources for people searching for naturopathic medicine, herbalism, homeopathy, acupuncture, and many other alternative therapies. Selfgrowth.com is one good resource that's a portal of sorts for alternative therapies. Although web sites and web site directories exist for just about any type of alternative therapy, there are some other jumping off points that may help you. Lyteforce.com provides links to Homeopathy Online, a helpful site that explains the concepts of dilutional therapy and other foundations of homeopathy, while providing resources for consumers interested in this form of medicine. Acupuncture.com is a similar resource. WholehealthMD.com is another site that provides a wealth of information.

Still, you must look out for alternative therapies that exploit the power of the Internet to lure you to their sites. In an earlier chapter, we discussed BreastCancer.com, a web site that clearly falls outside the conventions of modern medicine. No doubt you'd expect Menopause.com to provide information for women experiencing menopause. Instead, it points you toward alternative therapies, many of which contradict proven facts of modern gynecology. This kind of information can be both difficult for and dangerous to laypersons.

Fortunately, the Internet boasts many resources for policing and debunking alternative therapies. The National Council for Reliable Health Information (NCRHI.org) offers tools for you to identify responsible, reliable, evidence-driven health information. This site maintains lists of Internet charlatans, hucksters, and quacks. Another popular, useful site is Quackwatch.com. This site monitors the promotion of harmful health practices.

Keep these guidelines in mind when reviewing alternative medicine web sites.

1) Avoid sites that claim to improve your health or cure diseases based solely on nutritional supplements. Although some diseases are related to diet, most aren't.

2) Beware of testimonials. Many testimonials leave out important facts about conventional therapies. Some are complete fabrications.

3) Avoid sites that promise therapies where results can't be measured. This includes therapies that claim to detoxify you or balance your body's chemistries.

4) Stay away from sites that claim that the medical profession, drug companies, or the government oppose their therapies. It's illogical for anyone to oppose a medical therapy that might work, unless it's dangerous.

5) Similarly, keep away from any treatment that's touted as "secret." Methods that work are always widely publicized. Alternative therapies often aim to undermine your confidence in your doctor.

6) Check with your doctor before using herbal remedies. They may contain harmful byproducts and contaminants, or may have dangerous interactions with your regular prescription medicines.

7) Beware of any therapy that claims to be effective against a wide range of diseases or claims to be a cure-all.

8) Don't let desperation cloud your judgement. Incurable conditions may lead you to a controlled clinical trial. Don't seek out an alternative therapeutic solution that may make your situation worse.

9) Promoters of alternative therapies often use scientific terms and quote from the scientific literature.

Not all alternative therapy is quackery. Several useful conventional therapies started out as alternative practices. In 100 years, we may look back and say, "the cure for that disease was right in front of us!" For the present, however, I believe medical therapies should be rigorously scrutinized and subjected to scientific debate and review.

Discussion Groups and Chat Rooms

Online discussion groups, chat rooms, message boards, and forums let you reach other Internet users who share your interests. Chat rooms have sprouted up for a slew of medical conditions. They range from rooms for smoking cessation to those for rare immunodeficiencies. Such rooms exist on large medical web sites, alternative therapy sites, and even some doctor-and hospital-promoted web sites. In these rooms you'll find both people with genuine medical concerns and those who are simply looking for someone to talk to.

Often there are scheduled chat events, such as live interactions with experts on specific health topics. You and others attending the event may have a chance to ask questions.

People looking for someone to talk to are often willing to listen. Some people turn to chat rooms when they need emotional support. Although some chatters seek advice, many people enter chat rooms looking for validation of their medical complaints or treatment options.

Chat room participants often use pseudonyms to protect their privacy. This may protect your identity, but everyone who's logged in sees the thoughts you share. These rooms are intended for those seeking medical information, but they are freely accessible to anyone. Any information you disclose when posting a message becomes public.

Some participants in health care chat rooms have no interest in health care. They're simply interested in contacting others. Adults should monitor their children's chats. Discussion groups allow unscrupulous people to reach customers and potential victims. No legitimate practitioner will give out advice in a chat room, both for privacy and liability reasons. Be careful of what you type. Get the full credentials of anyone who offers you advice in a professional capacity.

The use of email discussion webs is a growing trend in discussion groups. There are now several groups where you can sign up and routinely receive emails that contain the group's discussions. You need not be an active participant in the discussion group to receive these emails. We've discussed the loss of privacy when using email. These discussion web emails may be subject to the same cookie-based technology as other Internet transmissions. Therefore, their privacy is in question. Moreover, users who post messages in a forum make their email available to others. You could receive unsolicited emails from third parties who see your email address on forwarded messages.

One chat room regular recently told me of a person who was waiting to hear about a hoped-for liver transplant. When the transplant didn't come through, that person received a lot of emotional support from the other chat room participants.

Patient Advocacy Groups

Patient advocacy groups are organizations of patients with a particular disease or condition. These groups provide assistance and psychological support for their members. Further, they are a vital link to others with similar conditions. In addition to patients, these groups usually include doctors, clergy, and political activists. Advocacy groups often lobby for reforms, research funds, and financial assistance for their members. There are individual web sites for almost every condition. Patientadvocacy.org is a general patient advocacy site. You can find more specialized sites for heart disease, Alzheimer's disease, or stroke.

Cancer advocacy sites are created along types of cancer or even types of treatments. For example, bonemarrow.org gives cancer patients information on treatment decisions and lobbying efforts, and provides links to appropriate web sites. These sites are resources for hard-to-find information and occasionally for good alternative therapy information. Many patient advocacy groups have consulting physicians who screen their site's contents.

Patient advocacy web sites are also important for consumers who can't get the treatment recommended by their doctors, because disputes about insurance coverage. Such disagreements usually involve complex contractual issues, which are typically difficult to resolve. Patient who are already seriously ill shouldn't be subjected to the additional stress of doing battle over insurance coverage. Many of these sites are familiar with these problems and have resources to help you.

You also can get help with your medical problems by finding pro-bono (free) legal advice and counsel, foreign language translation, and psychological counseling. Finally, patient advocacy groups can help you navigate the complexities and restrictions of managed care-based health delivery.

Overall, patient advocacy sites tend to be excellent starting points for your Internet health care research. Your only problem may be identifying the site that's most appropriate for your condition.

Clinical Trials

The Internet is an excellent tool for finding clinical trials. It pro-vides an organized resource for searching the vast array of sites where these trials are discussed. If you're interested in a clinical trial, learn as much as you can about it before you join. The Internet provides information on treatment-oriented trials, as well as trials for prevention, early detection, and quality of life, and stud-ies to evaluate ways to modify disease-causing behaviors like tobacco use.

Most clinical trials are carried out in steps called phases. Each phase is designed to find different information. Patients may be eli-gible for studies in different phases, depending on their general condition, the type and stage of their disease, and what therapy, if any, they have already had. Patients are seen regularly to determine the effects of the treatment. Treatment always stops if side effects become too severe. Although the early phases of a clinical trial are risky, there's a reason why a treatment enters a clinical trial: It has been extensively tested in the laboratory or in animal studies, and has been shown to be effective.

You can find generalized information about clinical trials at Pharminfo.com. This web site also contains links to many clinical trial centers, discussion groups, and clinical trial email services. You can also find a large list of clinical trials at Centerwatch.com. Look for trials specific to cancer at the National Cancer Institute's web site, NCI.NIH.gov.

Many medical web sites have information and links to clinical trials, as well as resources to match you to an appropriate trial. Researchers select subjects who are alike in certain ways, depending on the trial's purpose. Every protocol identifies specific characteristics the enrollees should have in order to participate in the study. These characteristics include age, type of disease and its stage, and general health. There are many web sites that guide you through eligibility criteria. Discuss your choices with your doctor and with those close to you.

You should be aware of some controversies regarding Internet access to clinical trials. Many investigators and patients dislike the advertising nature of clinical trials. Many links to clinical trials take the form of banner ads. Medical investigation is, after all, a business. Whether publicly or privately funded, it needs to attract patients. Clinical trial organizations and pharmaceutical companies now the Internet for patient recruitment.

Another drawback is that there's no single, reliable web site where consumers can compare all clinical trials and determine their best choices. Some investigators have set up comparative sites. Unfortunately, many of these are tainted by either a profit motive or deliberate misinformation.

Keep in mind the Internet security issues pertaining to information transmitted about clinical trials, especially the kind of communications that support the conduct of and convey the results of clinical trials. When entering any clinical trial, one of your key rights is the right to informed consent. Informed consent means that you must be given all the facts about a study before you to take part in it. This includes details about treatments and tests you may receive, and their possible benefits and risks. Gather as much information as possible about a clinical trial, and to take the time to understand it and weigh your possible benefits and risks.

Chapter 8.

Using Online Information for Health Insurance Concerns

According to Cyber Dialogue, an Internet market research firm, 78% of Internet users with health coverage say they're interested in managing their benefits through their insurance carrier's web site. Unfortunately, only 8% of these users actually use their insurer's web site. Sixty-eight percent aren't even aware that their insurer has a site.

Despite this growing interest, the insurance companies have been slow to move into the Internet marketplace. Most of these services aren't available online. One reason may be a deliberate decision to restrict the information available to their customers.

The nature of health insurance changed dramatically in the United States during the 1990s. Health care is now big business. It amounts to a huge percentage of the consumer dollars spent each year. The cost of health care has led many people to advocate universal health care access, price controls on medications, and medical savings accounts.

In 1992, there were serious proposals before Congress to create a federally run health care system. Many patients and most doctors opposed these proposals. In response, big business entered the health care marketplace. HMOs and other forms of managed care replaced traditional forms of indemnity and fee-for-service insurance plans. Managed care companies look at patients as customers. Costs are tightly controlled, medical treatments are carefully restricted, and doctors are paid a lot less for their services.

Most HMOs pay doctors a global capitated fee for a patient's yearly medical care. Your primary care doctor probably gets about $120.00 per patient per year, whether or not a patient actually sees the doctor or is hospitalized. In the past, HMO contracts often had gag clauses that kept doctors from discussing how managed care really works. Now that doctors are free of these restrictions, many patients are seeing the deficiencies of the HMO system and switching to other forms of insurance. Many doctors published articles on the Internet divulging the restrictions HMOs once held them to.

Superimposed on all these changes is the ever-present Internet. Although every insurance plan now has a web site, many of these sites provide little useful information. Some select sites may include up-to-date information on medical breakthroughs or therapies, especially if they are among the company's "accepted" or "recommended" practices. More typically, these sites include a health plan's patient education material in a carefully constructed format that may exclude important information.

Some insurance company and managed care web sites, however, can be excellent starting points for researching care guidelines, health care benefits, and in some cases, the dangers of unrestricted medical care. Your insurance company's web site should be one of your first stops. You may find that your benefits don't cover certain medical therapies. The site may also explain why your insurance company believes that a widely touted treatment is dangerous or too expensive. Sites such as AetnaUSHealthcare.com provide information on member health education as part of their preventive and wellness programs. Many sites allow you to search for participating doctors, as well.

Searching for a doctor on your insurance company or managed care provider's web site is far better than thumbing through a provider directory. Often the web site provides information such as an individual doctor's interests and specialties, office hours, and languages spoken.

Medicare.org lets you download documents that explain Medicare's benefits. Careful reading shows that Medicare restricts screening tests. Although the site says that routine screening is covered for many lab tests, this isn't true.

Some managed care sites, such as AetnaUShealthcare.com, Prudentialhealth.com, and Cigna.com, use confusing language to describe benefits. You might see a statement that certain tests may be available to you "after discussing the pros and cons of these tests with your doctor to determine if you are a candidate for screening." In many cases, though, managed care customers and Medicare recipients must either have active symptoms to justify the test, or must sign a statement that they will pay for the test.

You can see how companies use the Internet to present information so subtly that it doesn't seem like benefits are restricted. The take-home lesson is that managed care sites have vested interests, just like other companies that maintain sites. Review sites carefully and don't rely solely on this information.

Capitation is the reimbursement method almost all HMOs use. Doctors get a single fee for each patient, typically $8-10 per month per patient. This fee stays the same, whether the doctor sees the patient or not, whether the patient is hospitalized or just has an office visit. With such low reimbursements, doctors often urge HMO patients to use the Internet to view their HMO's restrictions.

For insurance companies, customers' increasing access to the Internet is a two-edged sword. While the Internet may improve communication, it gives customers access to a lot of previously unavailable information. The Internet can open the door to information your insurance company may not want you to have.

Understanding Insurance Company Drug Formularies

One major change in health care has been insurance company formularies. Formularies are the groups of medications customers are limited to by their insurance companies. These lists are the result of contracts between managed care plans and pharmaceutical manufacturers. These businesses use Preferred Pharmaceutical Management (PPM) companies as middlemen. A PPM runs your prescription plan. It makes money by negotiating contracts and profiling the prescription patterns of individual doctors.

Insurance companies like this system because they can negotiate large volume discounts on certain medications. Drug companies like the system because a drug that's on formulary is a guaranteed sale, with no competition. Furthermore, if a patient gets a prescription for a drug which isn't on formulary, the drug company can charge an unrestricted price.

The big losers are doctors and patients. Doctors have a terrible time keeping track of which drugs are on each company's formulary. As PPM contracts come and go, a doctor may have to switch an individual patient's medication several times a year. Patients lose out because they are often restricted to the cheapest and least effective drugs. Drugs with clear benefits, ranging from a high efficacy to a low side-effect profile, are restricted from patient use.

Many managed care plans offer step therapy indications. Patients may have to take a drug for several months, to see whether or not it works, before they can try an off-formulary drug. Some managed care organizations require pre-approval for many medications. You or your doctor must provide a lot of private information to the managed care plan to get their authorization for the non-formulary drug. Many sites have forms and other information on how to apply for these exceptions.

Most managed care sites list their formularies, including drugs that are available as part of a step therapy program. Formularies are available, for example on AetnaUShealthcare.com, Cigna.com, and KaiserPermanente.org. Sometimes this information is out of date, however. Docnote.com has pooled several formularies on one site. To compare formularies, however, you must go to each site and search on the medication you're interested in.

Drug formularies keep costs down by restricting which drugs you can receive. Sometimes it is in your best interest to go "off formulary" for a non-formulary drug with a clear benefit. Otherwise you may have to wait a long time for an appeal or special request.

Insurance Companies' Web Presences

Despite the seeming popularity of sites such as drkoop.com, many medical sites aren't making money for their owners. By the end of the year 2000, drkoop.com and similar sites may no longer exist. Insurance company sites will rush in to fill this gap. This seems like a logical step, since insurance companies already provide medical information for their customers. The problem is that these companies have a vested interest in what you read on the Internet.

In my survey of the sites of the largest insurance companies (including AetnaUSHealthcare, Prudential, Cigna, Kaiser, and others), I found that each typically delivers:

1) patient educational material

2) drug formulary information

3) information for employers

4) online enrollment

5) selection information for doctors and health care providers

Many insurance company web sites have online forms for filing claims, filing appeals, and making special requests for medications. Again, be careful what type of information you transmit. At present, insurance company sites seem to be chiefly interested in providing an easy means for patient contact. One site, Cigna.com, includes a wealth of medical information, similar to the large commercial medical web sites. At this time, it is unclear whether these sites use cookies. In the future these sites may use online advertising to support the heavy traffic on them.

Some sites for insurance companies and managed care plans contain information about patient assistance programs. Many plans have special treatment services for asthma management, diabetes care, and heart disease. These treatment programs often offer integrated care—medical, dietary, and physical therapy support—all under the roof of your health plan. Managed care companies are spearheading efforts to use the Internet to integrate care for long-term diseases. The Internet is an excellent resource for discovering and evaluating these programs. It also provides a medium where patients can compare their treatment with that of others, perhaps eliminating any disparities in medical care.

A comprehensive list of health plans, sorted by state, can be found at Healthplans.com, which lists health plan web site addresses as well. This site also gives you health insurance cost and benefit comparisons. Many other insurance brokers maintain web sites with similar information.

Claim Denials—What You Can Do Online

One way that an insurance plan or managed care plan saves money is by denying claims. This may be the appropriate action in some cases, but patients have the right to appeal the decision. Insure.com is an excellent resource for information on claim denials. It provides information on what to do, online or off, if a claim is denied. Here are some general rules.

    1) The reason for denial should be stated on your explanation of benefits.

2) If you disagree with the denial, check your policy or employee booklet for the company's appeal procedures

3) Your appeal should be in writing and may require information from your doctor.

Few insurance companies allow appeals over the Internet. Some plans let you check the status of your claim online. Almost all of the large health plans let you print out denial claim forms on their web site. And of course, you can always email questions or comments to your health insurers. Just don't count getting an answer.

If you encounter a claim denial, an external review might help. This is a process you initiate. It subjects your claim to review by an auditor from outside of the insurance company. Some health insurance sites let you download documents to initiate the external review process. Lawyers specializing in claim denial litigation have their own web sites. Also there are advocacy group sites that can help you with claim denials and issues relating to coverage. You can gain more information by visiting or. An excellent page with links to many patient advocacy web sits can be found at the. Another good informational page on getting your managed care company to pay for your coverage can be found at. Your insurance company's site probably has useful information on how to appeal a claim denial. At least for now, though, it's best to make your appeal directly, and in writing.

Obviously insurance companies and managed care plans have far to go before they are full-service e-commerce entities. Privacy concerns notwithstanding, many Internet users would like to manage their health benefits through their insurance carrier's web sites. At this point, insurance company web sites generally do not allow sophisticated interactions such as online appeals of claim denials. They do, however, have some resources that you may find helpful.

Chapter 9.

What Online Practitioners Can and Should Offer

The ethical and legal implications of online medical care fall into four categories.

1) Confidentiality—Instantaneous access to medical records may be beneficial to the medical community, but it requires large databases that contain all of a patient's information. If these databases aren't properly protected, the confidentiality of medical records could be jeopardized.

2) Liability—Internet-based medical practice spreads liability if more than one doctor provides care. Conflicting jurisdictions may have conflicting malpractice laws.

3) Licensing—Medical licenses are issued by each state in the United States. It's illegal for a doctor to practice in a state where he or she isn't licensed.

4) Fraud—Identities can be falsified over the Internet. Anyone can impersonate a doctor.

Will the Internet progress from an excellent health research tool to a destination for personal health care? I doubt it. Nothing can replace a physical exam for making an accurate diagnosis. Doctors must use additional interpretive skills beyond hearing what the patient sees. They must use their powers of observation in conjunction with medical histories. This may mean being aware of subtle physical changes in body language, gait, or hair thickness, for example.

Among the problems with Internet-based medical care are:

1) There is no examination of the patient to determine if there is a medical problem and determine a specific diagnosis.
2) There is no dialogue with the patient to discuss treatment alternatives and to determine the best course of treatment.
3) There is no attempt to establish a reliable medical history.
4) There is no provision of information about the benefits and risks of the prescribed medication.
5) There is no follow-up to assess the therapeutic outcome.

Still, online medical care continues to grow in many arenas. Doctors offer advice in chat rooms. Consumers can participate in online medical conferences. Many large medical sites have doctors on staff to answer submitted questions and also to lead discussion forums. But these forms of doctor-patient contact lack one vital component of medical care—person-to-person contact.

Remote medical care is no replacement for the personal contact between a doctor and a patient. Examinations without these crucial human contacts can lead to misdiagnoses or delayed diagnoses. Delayed diagnosis is the chief fear listed in the American Medical Association's report on Internet-based medical practice (Report of the Board of Trustees, 35-A-99; American Medical Asssocation Annual Report 1999)

Computer-based Remote Medical Care-Telemedicine

Despite lacking important components, telemedicine is becoming more common. It can mean anything from calling your doctor for an antibiotic when you're away on a trip to using a special device that lets your doctor to examine you from afar. While this method of medical care is convenient, the critical parts of the doctor-patient relationship—touch and observation—are absent.

When doctors consult each other via video, email, telephone, or other technological means, they practice telemedicine. One of the goals of WebMD.com is the growth of this form of medical communication. Telemedicine can also be used for diagnosis or educational purposes. For example, a doctor can communicate with a patient or doctor in a remote area to aid in a diagnosis. Surgeons can watch procedures being done by other doctors and contribute their knowledge. Telemedicine can make a difference for patients in rural areas, whose nearest doctor may be miles away.

You can see how the Internet is a natural medium for these kinds of interactions. Among the potential benefits of telemedicine are an improvements in efficiency and convenience, reduced costs, and easier monitoring of patients.

Telemedicine is the use of electronic communication technologies to provide clinical care at a distance. We may think of telemedicine as a sophisticated electronic interaction, but technically when your doctor gives advice by phone, he or she is practicing telemedicine. Telemedicine may increasingly come to mean having an online doctor whom you've never met, as well as an online pharmacy. The next step is to connect the physician with the pharmacy and do everything online—from diagnosis to filling your prescription.

Web Prescriptions

Online pharmacies have the same medical and legal issues as online doctoring. Every state licenses its pharmacists. When prescription are filled via the Internet, a pharmacist may fill orders for a person from a state where he or she is not licensed to dispense. Some states are beginning to approve this type of interstate pharmacy practice. But international pharmacy sites pose another danger. People can buy drugs that aren't approved for use in the United States.

We will discuss buying medications prescribed during a face-to-face visit with your doctor in the next chapter. Just remember, there's a big difference between getting a prescription filled online, and getting a medication prescribed online.

There are several web sites where consumers can buy medications without seeing a doctor. Many such sites are serviced by physicians who prescribe and dispense medications. Most Internet prescribing has centered on sidenafil (Viagra), a prescription drug used to treat erectile dysfunction. There are now hundreds of sites where you can get this medication without seeing a doctor. One such site, Net-Dr.com, lets you buy drugs for erectile dysfunction, hair loss, weight loss, and arthritis. All of these drugs have potential side effects. Purchaser must waive liability and fill out a short health questionnaire. The site has doctors on its payroll, who review the questionnaires. Once a doctor approves your questionnaire, the company sends you the medicines you ordered.

In the case of Viagra™, the questionnaire asks purchasers about a history of heart disease or their regular medications—known contraindications to taking this drug. What the questionnaires don't ask about are other symptoms. This uncollected information might lead a doctor to a diagnosis of diabetes or a pituitary tumor—common causes of erectile dysfunction. Masking this important symptom can lead to deadly consequences.

Under the existing laws of most states, prescribing drugs to patients outside the state where the physician is licensed is considered the unlicensed practice of medicine. Additionally, every state's medical board agrees that issuing prescriptions without performing a physical exam or reviewing patients' medical records is practicing an unacceptable level of medical care. As of the year 2000, there are no federal laws regulating Internet prescribing or Internet medical practice. Some states, however, have bills that include diagnosis and transfer of medical information "through electronic means" in their definition of "practicing medicine," regardless of whether or not the patient and doctor are in the same state.

Another large problem on the Internet is foreign based pharmacy web sites. Some of these sites illegally promote and distribute unapproved and approved prescription drugs in the United States. Typically, these companies post price lists and advertise U.S.-patented prescription drugs at greatly reduced prices. In some cases, the ads state that drugs can be ordered without a prescription.

The illegal distribution of drugs from foreign sources raises concerns over the quality of these drugs and whether patients are at risk due to lack of physician oversight or inadequate directions for use. The Food and Drug Administration has had little success regulating this trade.

If you plan to order medications online, without seeing your doctor, consider these issues:

1) Web sites that prescribe medications without doctors' prescriptions are more likely to attract patients who might lie about their medical histories.

2) The Internet environment meant that patients aren't able to judge the qualifications of the person making the online prescription.

3) There are few, if any, standards for online pharmacies or web sites.

4) Prescription web sites circumvent laws that exist to protect the public from dangerous products.

I believe that patients should only get prescriptions from their personal physicians, never from online physicians hired just to write prescriptions. Getting a prescription drug by filling out a questionnaire can pose serious health risks. A questionnaire doesn't give a doctor enough information about you. Ideally, a doctor should be able to tell whether a drug is safe for you or safe to use, whether another treatment is more appropriate, or whether you have an underlying medical condition that would make using that drug may be harmful.

Getting a prescription from an unknown doctor online may include risks of misdiagnosis, wrong dosing, and drug interaction. If a site does not require a patient to have a prescription for medication, the potential exists for mistakes. An unscrupulous online pharmacy might send the wrong medication. There would be little recourse in such a situation.

Viagra is a registered trademark of Pfizer Pharmaceuticals

Chapter 10.

Purchasing Drugs and Other Health Care Products Online

The option to purchase health care products and pharmaceuticals online is a natural outgrowth of the explosion in online consumerism. The Internet may be the greatest medium for delivering pharmaceutical information. Direct appeals to end users clearly pay off. Some people already ask their doctors for prescription medicines by name. Pharmaceutical advertisers focus almost all of their efforts on Internet exposure of their medications. Traditional brick and mortar pharmacies are establishing online presences.

Most people turn to these resources for convenience and cost—no waiting in long lines, no large prices. Actually, prices at online pharmacies aren't always lower than those at traditional pharmacies, but the Internet lets you make a valid price comparison. A 1999 survey by *Consumer Reports* showed that buyers could save as much as 29 percent by getting certain drugs online.

Most online pharmacies offer different services than your neighborhood pharmacy. Traditionally, neighborhood pharmacies were places for consultation and advice. Your pharmacist might suggest medications for you. Unfortunately, small pharmacies have given way to large chain pharmacies. Encounters between customers and trained pharmacists are less common. The host of informational services online pharmacies provide may make up for this loss of service.

1) How long will medications be prescribed for you?

2) How will this medication help me?

3) What are the side effects of this medicine?

4) Are there any medicines I should avoid while taking this medication?

Online pharmacies are particularly effective at helping you answer these questions. This is especially important if you're taking several medicines, because the side effects of medications rise exponentially the more medications you take.

Perhaps the chief attractions of purchasing medications online are the speed and ease of choosing and ordering products. Moreover, online pharmacies can give customers product information and references to other sources of information much more easily than traditional pharmacies. As the computer technology that allows doctors to transmit prescriptions to pharmacies expands, we should see a reduction in prescription errors. Finally, many online pharmacies can email you with reminders that your prescription is about to run out.

Here are some important guidelines for ordering from online pharmacies.

1) Plan ahead. Online pharmacies send your medications by mail. Although some companies offer rush service, you should figure on at least a day between when you send in your prescription and when you receive your medications. Keep a small supply of medicine on hand to cover this period.

2) Have your information ready. Online pharmacies typically need a copy of the prescription, your physician's phone number, your insurance information, and a credit card number.

3) Comparison-shop. Many online pharmacies offer significant discounts over traditional pharmacies. However, you may be billed a dispensing fee and shipping charges.

4) Rely on customer service. Most online pharmacies provide excellent customer service where you can access
instant order tracking

The advantages of online pharmacies may include lower prices
and easier availability of drugs. The latter is especially true for those
for whom a trip to the pharmacy can be difficult and people who
live far from a pharmacy.

Medications Online

If your doctor writes you a prescription for a week's worth of
antibiotics, it's probably not worth going to an online pharmacy.
The delay in starting your medication could be inconvenient and
even dangerous. Most medications sold, however, are for long-term
use—usually for the lifetime of the patient. These medications treat
incurable yet treatable conditions such as diabetes, hypertension,
heart disease, and AIDS. People on long-term medications have
used mail-order medication suppliers and pharmacies for years.
Online pharmacies are simply an extension of this service. If your
medication costs run into thousands of dollars a year, online pharmacies may offer you significant savings.

Patients who take long-term medications are just the people
pharmaceutical manufacturers and advertisers target. Patients who
switch from one company's blood pressure medication to another's
might add up to thousands of dollars of profit. That's why pharmaceutical manufacturers and advertisers are intensely interested in
the consumer habits of long-term medication users. That's why
they're putting more ads on pharmaceutical web sites. They hope
you'll ask your doctor to change your medicine—to their medicine.
Among my patients, those who get drug information from the
Internet are much more likely to request brand-name drugs.

Here are some guidelines to use when purchasing medications online.

1) Check with the National Association of Boards of Pharmacy website, www.nabp.com. if the site is a licensed pharmacy in good standing. Don't buy from sites that offer to prescribe a prescription drugs for the first time without a physical exam, sell a prescription drug without a prescription, or sell drugs not approved by FDA.

2) Make sure the pharmacy web site provides access to a registered pharmacist to answer questions.

3) Confirm that the pharmacy web site has a United States address and a phone number to call if there's a problem.

4) Beware of sites that advertise a "new cure" for a serious disorder or a quick cure-all for a wide range of ailments.

5) Beware of sites that use impressive-sounding terminology to disguise a lack of good science, or those that claim the government, the medical profession, or research scientists have conspired to suppress their product.

6) Avoid sites that include undocumented case histories, such as patient testimonials.

7) Talk to your health-care professional before using any medication for the first time.

Advertising Medications Online

Online pharmacies certainly use cookie technology and online advertisements. When you make a purchase, they collect your credit card information as well as other demographic information. As we discussed in earlier chapters, this information is used to profile you for marketing purposes.

The FDA and Federal Trade Commission do, in part, regulate ads on the Internet. Ads for FDA-approved drugs must be accompanied by information on side effects, safety, and efficacy. There are, however, many non-FDA products advertised on these sites. The FDA also regulates the actual prescribing process and ensures that drugs aren't sold without proper prescriptions. Though these are still fairly new regulatory responsibilities, the FDA has already successfully shut down sites involved in illegal trade.

Unfortunately, on the Internet it's easy for the unscrupulous to get around the FDA's safeguards. Web sites may misrepresent themselves as affiliates of legitimate pharmacies. In a report to the FDA, the Center for Drug Evaluation and Research raised significant concerns about the Internet's difficulties for the regulators, law enforcement agencies, and policymakers that protect public health and safety.

"A significant public health risk exists when a consumer is at risk for harm (1) from the use of the product, (2) as the result of not taking approved drugs for a specific disease or condition, or (3) by delaying medical treatment recognized as safe and effective for a specific disease or condition."

Don't turn to online pharmacies for non-FDA-approved foreign medicines. It's illegal to import such drugs into the United States. The FDA's personal importation policy does, however, allow you to bring in an unapproved drug for personal use for a serious condition, providing there has been no promotion of the drug to U.S. residents. Additional information is available at www.fda.gov.

Many online pharmacies contain ads for unapproved new drugs (including counterfeit drugs), for products based on fraudulent health claims, and for non-prescription medications. According to the FDA, bodybuilding and exercise-related nutritional supplements are among the most common of these heavily marketed products.

Finding More Information

One advantage of online pharmacies is that you can print out information on potential drug side effects and drug interactions. PlanetRx.com and drkoop.com offer excellent drug interaction information. In addition to researching infinite medication interactions, you can analyze over-the-counter products and even food items. Additional food and drug interactions can be found at foodmedinteractions.com.

RxList.com is another interesting and important resource. This web site lets you enter the imprint information from a pill to figure out which pill it is. This may be invaluable in an emergency situation such as trying to help someone who's unconscious.

Although the information provided by these and similar sites is purely informational, it may sometimes catch a potentially dangerous interaction your doctor might have overlooked. Most of these sites make you agree to a waiver of responsibility before using them to gather drug information. This minimizes the site's liability in case you take the wrong medicine or take a medication in the wrong way.

Many pharmacy web sites are the first places where you'll find newly released medications and hard-to-find medications. Because these online pharmacies sell the newest medications, their web sites may be excellent places to learn of new information on changes of treatment guidelines. For example, the treatment of HIV changes on an almost monthly basis. Many HIV patients must take several costly medications at once. Waiting in line at their local pharmacy is too time consuming. Often, HIV patients report that the newest medications aren't available or are back-ordered in these establishments. Many online pharmacies can get these medications right away, and can also inform patients about new medication releases, medication changes, and withdrawals from the market.

It's important for you to track information on a medication release or withdrawal. The FDA's drug review process has been streamlined in recent years, resulting in significantly reduced review times. As a result, many drugs have made it to market before being adequately tested. Many physicians have been all too willing to prescribe these new drugs. Since 1998, many widely prescribed medications have been withdrawn from the market because of serious and sometimes deadly side effects. Many online pharmacies and other medical web sites contribute to post-marketing surveillance of a drug by allowing you or your doctor to report any problems.

Drug interactions occur when a medicine reacts with other medicines or with the foods you eat. Prescription drugs, nonprescription medicines, and vitamins are all subject to interactions. Some interactions can be harmful to your health or reduce the effectiveness of a drug. When you input a medication on most pharmacy web sites, you will be given information on cost, directions for use, side effects, and correct dosage. This information is significantly more extensive than what you get at a "brick and mortar" pharmacy and usually very well organized. Pharmacy web sites are usually the first places to notify you if a drug is withdrawn from the market or restricted in use.

Alternative Health Products for Sale

Online pharmacies don't just sell prescription medications. Like their brick-and-mortar counterparts, these companies sell products from diapers to shampoo. These items are also available by mail order. Convenience is the chief advantage of buying such items through the Internet. Prices aren't necessarily cheaper, and you pay for shipping. Despite this, online pharmacies report brisk sales of their non-medication offerings.

Also available from online pharmacies are alternative health products, including vitamins, antioxidants, and homeopathy supplements. The Naturalpharmacist.com is an excellent source for non-prescription nutritional products, herbs, and supplements. This web site claims to provide unbiased, medically relevant information on its products. It has a large searchable database for supplement interactions, plus an interactive tool to determine whether a particular supplement is right for you.

Wholehealthmd.com combines conventional medicine and alternative nutritional products. This site specializes in nutritional supplements and has a database relating diet and nutrition to many common diseases. Several of these alternative product web sites have newsletters and email services to keep you updated on new products.

When purchasing alternative products, keep in mind potential interactions with prescription medications you take. Also be aware of the danger of receiving tainted or dangerous products that aren't overseen by the FDA. Rx.com has an important resource for researching interactions between prescription medications and alternative health products. This site has a searchable *Physicians' Desk Reference*—the textbook most doctors refer to when writing prescriptions. In addition, the site has an online home reference database for herbs and natural remedies. Another site, Healthquick.com, provides a searchable database of herbs and herbal remedies, including plant descriptions, precautions, and possible interactions.

In my practice, I find that many patients actively seek alternative medical products. This may be due to dissatisfaction with traditional medical care or merely a willingness to try something new. Media attention and exposure may contribute to the growing interest in these products. I often steer my patients to some of the sites I've described, after providing appropriate precautions. One site, Thriveonline.com partners with Oxygen.com, a woman-oriented web site. Patients who have used this site tell me that they found reasonable and rational information on medical-nutritional integration.

The Internet is closing the gap between traditional and alternative medicine. Equal access to alternative medicine and alternative medical products, for both doctors and patients, guarantees that many of these therapies will be integrated into traditional medical practice. In addition, many commonly used alternative therapies will be debunked when subjected to scrutiny.

Many sites sell products that combine conventional medicine with alternative therapies, in an attempt for the body to strengthen and heal itself. Doctors are increasingly integrating these products into their medical repertoire.

About the Author

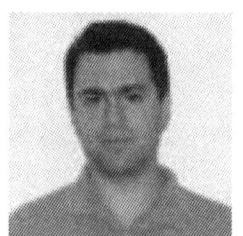 Dr. Kroll is an Assistant Professor of Medicine at Georgetown University Medical Center. He has been involved in teaching concepts about on-line health information to medical students for several years. He is also involved in creating tools to streamline use of the web for physicians. He has been long—been involved in web-based research, having set up a on-line research system for genetics and molecular biology more than 10 years ago. Dr. Kroll is board certified in Internal Medicine and holds a Ph.D. in Clinical pharmacology. Most importantly, he has no vested interests or ties to any online companies, pharmaceutical companies or other such interests.

Appendix A—Chapter Quizzes

Chapter 1 Quiz
  1. What is the traditional method of medical data validation?
  A) Peer review by competitors.
  B) Television broadcast.
  C) Pre-released summaries of important findings.
  D) Publishing on the Internet.

  2. Which is not a method of generating "hype" around a medical discovery?
  A) Directed E-mail.
  B) Promotion as a "medical update."
  C) Attaching a physician's name to the discovery.
  D) Comparing it to similar findings.

  3. How many medically oriented websites are there currently estimated to be?
  A) 5000
  B) 12000
  C) 18000
  D) 25000

  4. What is a portal?
  A) A place for a ship to dock.
  B) A search engine oriented website.
  C) A method of Internet privacy.
  D) An letter generated by E-mail.

5. What can't you learn from an Online Pharmacy Website?
A) drug interactions.
B) new drug formulations.
C) alternative therapies.
D) pharmaceutical companies profits.

6. What can't the Internet do for you?
A) A physical examination.
B) Ask you about symptoms.
C) Take your medical history.
D) Offer medical advice.

7. What don't websites do with your registration information?
A) Sell it to advertisers.
B) E-mail you a response.
C) Link it to your activity on the website.
D) Throw it out.

8. What method should you use for navigating the Internet?
A) Give away as much information as possible.
B) Ignore information from large medical websites.
C) Limit your search to cures for cancer.
D) Discuss your research with your doctor.

9. True or False? Why are people turning to the Internet for health information?
A) A second opinion.
B) Less time spent with their doctor.
C) The speed by which medical information is posted.
D) They are required by their insurance company.
E) They want to bypass medical school.

10. True or False? How do some medical information websites make money?

A) Advertising revenue.
B) Pharmaceutical company grants.
C) Referrals to other commercial websites.
D) Selling products.
E) Registered customer lists.

Chapter 1 Answer Key

1) Correct answer A. Traditional forms of data validation occur by peer review. In a typical case, a researcher will send the paper which he wrote to a journal. The editors of that journal will in turn send the paper to other resarchers in the field for review. Often these are direct competitors. These reviewers will comment on the paper, and determine whether it is suitable for publication. Other forms of information release, which we encounter everyday, undermine this peer review process. These include broadcasting data on television or the internet as well as the pre-release of information before publication.

2) Correct Answer D. Medical information is often "hyped" to generate interest. The Internet has increased the likelihood of this by adding new methods for disseminating information. Directed E-mail is one of these new methods. Medical updates are very often posted on websites to get a readers attention. This is simply a marketing tool. Additionally, attaching a physician's name to a discovery lends credibility to that discovery and can be used for indexing purposes on the Internet.

3) Correct Answer C. And this is growing every day.

4) Correct Answer B. Portals are entry points to the Internet. A portal's search engine is where most people start their information gathering. Cookies technology is a controvertial method which may undermine Internet privacy. A letter which is mass emailed is called SPAM.

5) Correct Answer D. Pharmaceutical company profits are not generally publicized. A lot of useful information is available on Pharmacy websites including drug interactions, new drug formulations and alternative therapies. Remember, however, that these websites are in the business of selling pharmaceutical products.

6) Correct Answer A. Resources on the Internet can substitute for a physician's skills in many ways. Many websites are sophisticated in terms of the questions they ask and the decision trees that they use. A physician's examination also involves a decision tree based upon findings. No website can substitute for examination by a physician.

7) Correct Answer D. Registration information is amongst the most valuable resources that a Website can attain. This information can be used to profile you demographically for advertisors. This demographic information can be supplemented by a record of your website activity. The websites use your registration information to communicate with you.

8) Correct Answer D. Always discuss all your findings with your doctor before acting on Internet research. There is no substitute for medical training and certification. Never give away a lot of information about yourself on the Internet. Many of the large websites have scrutinized and screened information from smaller websites and are thus an excellent resource for your research. There is no one single cure for cancer. Cancer patients should be realistic when using the Internet and try to find safe and effective methods of treatment.

9) Correct Answers True,True,True,False,False People are turning to the Internet for a variety of reasons. At this point, no insurance company requires you to be connected to the Internet. Although many people want to gather information, it

is not reasonable to say that people want to bypass traditional medical training.

10) Correct Answers True, True, True, True, True There are many ways for websites to make money. Medical information websites also use some specific consumer health methods.

Chapter 2 Quiz

1. Which method will improve your medical search?
A) Try alternate spellings of your search terms.
B) Restrict your search to American-only publications.
C) Type as many words as possible into the search engine.
D) Put important words in capitals.

2. What is the Boolean method?
A) A school of psychiatry.
B) A method of searching based on logical mathematical principles.
C) A method of ranking search results.
D) A process of physical therapy after a motor vehicle accident.

3. Which operator is not commonly found in search engines?
A) And
B) Or
C) Not
D) Who

4. What is a META tag?
A) A method of indexing a web page for a search engine.
B) A tag on a bottle of pills.
C) A very large advertisement.
D) An index used by pharmaceutical companies to find patients.

5. Which of the following is correct about the medical journal database at the NIH?
A) It is free to all users.

B) It contains all medical journals published.

C) It is the last place you should check in your health research.

D) It is not recommended by doctors.

6. Using the Search Phrase "Liver AND Cirrhosis NOT Alcohol" will yield which results?

A) All web pages or articles on the liver and cirrhosis.

B) Those that contain the words liver and cirrhosis, but not those that also contain the word alcohol.

C) Web pages that contain the words liver and alcohol but not the word cirrhosis.

D) Web pages that contain the words cirrhosis but not those that contain the word liver.

7. Which of the following is a widely read medical journal?

A) Bob's Orthopedic Weekly.

B) The Magna Carta.

C) The Cambodian Journal of Neurology.

D) The New England Journal of Medicine.

8.What is the website BreastCancer.com?

A) An informative site for conventional chemotherapy.

B) An alternative natural medicine website.

C) A link to the bone marrow transplant donors' website.

D) A portal for searching the Internet for breast cancer information.

9.What is a spider?

A) An arachnid with 6 legs.

B) A method that a search engine uses for indexing WebPages.

C) A search term generator for search engines.

D) A method for linking websites together.

10. True or False? The search term "Heart*" will yield which results

A) All web pages or articles with the word "heart."
B) All with the phrase "Hearty appetite."
C) All with the word "Heartburn."
D) All with the phrase "Heat stroke."
E) All with the word "Hearing."

Chapter 2 Answer Key

1) Correct Answer A. Alternate spellings of words may be important. Many websites are indexed by words in their titles. Restricting your search to a specific country or language will limit the scope of your search. Typing as may words as possible may cause too restrictive a search. Search engines are usually case insensitive—meaning that capital letters are not required.

2) Correct Answer B. Boolean searches entail using search terms and conjunctions such as AND or OR to find a logical set of search results. The search terms are typically ranked according to relevancy.

3) Correct Answer D. Who is not a Boolean operator, although some search engines, including the National Library of Medicine allow you to input the term AU=xyz, where xyz is an author name. And, Or and Not are powerful Boolean operators that can significantly improve the quality of your search.

4) Correct Answer A. META tags are embedded words and phrases that the web user cannot directly see when reading a web page. These META tags are used to index a web page. Advertisements on the Internet are usually in the form of banner ads. These banner ads are placed on web pages. Pharmaceutical companies keep careful records of which patients are taking certain drugs. These records are not called META tags.

5) Correct Answer A. Medline and the National Library of Medicine is free to all users. Although it contains thousands of

medical journals in hundreds of languages, it does not contain all published medical journals. It should often be the first place to check when initiating health research, because the medical literature can lead you to correct search terms, relevant researchers and up-to-date information. Most doctors use this resource as a primary source of research information.

6) Correct Answer B. Using the Boolean operators AND and NOT will yield a conjunction of the first two search terms with the exclusion of all results that contain the third search term.

7) Correct Answer D. The New England Journal of Medicine is the most widely read medical journal in the world. Many journals are disseminated free to readers and are known as "throw—away" publications. These journals often solicit articles from researchers, rather than restricting published articles to peer reviewed scrutiny.

8) Correct Answer B. BreastCancer.com is one of the many names that were gobbled up during the rush to register website names. Many of these are now being used to obscure information and confuse consumers. Never start your research by simply adding .com to end of your condition.

9) Correct Answer B. Many search engines use spiders as a tool to "crawl" through the entire World Wide Web and index all pages. Other spiders are sent out deliberately to index a particular web page. Search term generators exist for some search engines to assist you with a search. Arachnids have 8 legs. Although spiders typically spin webs, websites are not linked together by spiders.

10) Correct Answers True, True, True ,False, False Truncating a word with a * at the end will give ALL results with the letters before the * and any letters after. Heat stroke and Hearing do not contain the letters of Heart. Hearty appetite and Heartburn do contain the letters of Heart.

Chapter 3 Quiz
1) Which things are of value to an Internet company?
A) The number of "hits" to their website.
B) Their customer base.
C) The personal profiles that are built around you.
D) all of the above.

2. Firewalls exist to:
A) protect your computer from combustion.
B) protect privacy.
C) shield surfers from being "cookied."
D) keep track of surfing history.

3. Many doctors offices already transmit what type of information by computer?
A) *insurance claims.*
B) chart notes.
C) doctor correspondence.
D) prescriptions.

4. What type of information is safe to transmit over the Internet?
A) your hair color.
B) your social security number.
C) your credit card number.
D) your address.

5. Internet Private Policy Statements are:
A) regulated by the FCC.
B) proof that a medical website is secure.
C) sometimes placed by the same people who want your information.
D) An agreement between you and your doctor.

6. Which statement most likely represents a legitimate medical claim?

A) Medical breakthrough.

B) University sponsored research.

C) Miracle cure.

D) Exclusive product.

7. Medical SPAM is:

A) An unsolicited health related e-mail.

B) An e-mail from your doctor.

C) Information found on medical websites.

D) Federally regulated.

8) Return Receipts are:

A) A method for SPAMers to track effectiveness.

B) The way the website knows you have returned for more information.

C) An e-mail from the post office.

D) A method for generating interest in a website.

9. True or False What items can a cookie contain?

A) Passwords.

B) The name of the website that you surfed from.

C) Credit card information.

D) A user name.

E) your web browser.

10. True or False?

A) Medical websites are typically non-profit entities

B) Most Medical websites are designed to give you non-biased information

C) There are no advertisements on The National Institutes of Health Website.

D) You should always attempt to surf the web anonymously for health care information.

E) You cannot erase the cookies from your computer.

Chapter 3 Answer Key

1) Correct Answer D. Web traffic, a large customer base or a defined customer base (i.e. all doctors or all lawyers), and personal profiles based upon your web surfing are all very valuable to an Internet company.

2) Correct Answer B. Firewalls are secure web-based servers that are set up around "intranets" that exist within companies. They are not like a firewall in your car which protects the passengers from an engine fire. They often do not protect users from being cookied. Cookies keep track of surfing history.

3) Correct Answer A. Doctors have used computers for many years to send insurance claims. Other forms of patient information, such as chart notes, doctor correspondence and prescriptions are increasingly being transmitted by computer, but only by a small number of doctors' offices.

4) Correct Answer A. You should never transmit anything over the Internet unless you are sure that no one else has access. This is even true in supposed secure socket layer (SSL) technology. Hackers have the ability to peek at this information. You should thin carefully before transmitting any information that may profile you or reveal private information.

5) Correct Answer C. Private policy statements are completely unregulated. Although they look nice, they provide no proof that a medical website is secure. Many of the groups that create this statements and certifications are the same groups that seek to gather your information. Your doctor and you should make an agreement about what information can be communicated over the Internet. This will be covered in a latter chapter.

6) Correct Answer B. University sponsored research has at least an air of credibility. It implies professional researchers at a university using funds that may have been obtained through a grant. Medical breakthroughs, miracle cures, exclusive products and secret ingredients are all promotional catch-phrases.

7) Correct Answer A. SPAM is the unsolicited e-mail that can clog your mailbox. Many mail servers allow you to block SPAM receipt from certain senders. The senders, however have some sophisticated ways of getting around this. E-mails from your doctor are usually solicited. SPAM is never federally regulated.

8) Correct Answer A. SPAMers use return receipts to tell if you have received and read an e-mail. Web sites track your activity, including your return activity by Cookie technology. The post office does not generally send e-mail, and may ultimately be replaced by e-mail. There are a lot of ways of generating interest in a website, including SPAM. Return receipts are not one of them.

9) Correct Answers True, True, True, True, True. Cookies have the ability to track all kinds of hidden and seemingly encrypted information.

10) Correct Answers False, False, True, True, True Most medical websites are profit motivated businesses. Most of the information they provide is sponsored or linked to advertisement and thus biased. The NIH websites have no advertisements as they are a government funded not-for-profit entity. When you Surf for health care information, if not done exclusively in an anonymous fashion, you should at least pay attention to privacy issues. Cookies can be erased from your computer. There is generally a Cookie folder in your System or Windows folders.

Chapter 4 Quiz

1) Treatment decision tools are:

A) online assistants for searching the medical web.

B) large databases of doctor managed patient files

C) available on all medical websites

D) interactive disease management resources .

2) The Health Information Portability and Accountability Act:

A) Is an act by the US Congress to allow you to carry around your own medical records.

B) Allows many different types of interested parties access to your health information.

C) Generally viewed by doctors as a significant improvement in privacy issues.

D) does not require standardization of medical records.

3) Who generally may not have access to your medical records based upon your signed waiver when you initiated health insurance coverage?

A) your employer

B) your insurance company

C) the federal government

D) The Internal Revenue Service

4) Which of the following is true about maintaining your medical records online?

A) You can upload your own x-rays.

B) You cannot specify who has access to your online medical records

C) You cannot enter medication information.

D) Programs can remind you of important dates for health prevention.

5) SPAM e-mails should never contain:

A) Advertisements for products

B) Useful information.

C) Your credit card information.

D) Hyperlinks to relevant information.

6) When you register at a medical website:

A) You may sign up for medically related email

B) Your email address is inserted into the websites mailing list

C) Your email address and other demographic information may be sold to an advertiser

D) All of the above

7) Blood pressure tracking programs on the Internet

A) Can take your blood pressure via your computer.

B) Track your blood pressure, based upon the numbers you input.

C) Recommend specific medications

D) Send your information to your doctor.

8) True or False? Surveys on Medical websites often lead to:

A) you receiving targeted e-mail

B) information being sold to advertisers

C) poll results being posted for public viewing

D) Promotional banner advertisement delivery

E) Restricted areas of the medical website for viewing.

9) True or False? A Doctors access to your patient chart:

A) Can make the difference in a life or death situation

B) Is restricted according to your wishes.

C) Is increasingly occurring over the Internet.

D) Is private and secure on the Internet.

E) Permits doctors to transfer your care when you move.

Chapter 4 Answer Key

1) Correct Answer D. Treatment decision tools are only available on some medical websites. They are designed to give you an interactive tool for managing your illness. Questions such as severity, duration of time, and quality of symptoms might be asked. There are online assistant programs for assisting you in searching the medical web.. These can be found at Yahoohealth.com, for example. Large databases of patient files are maintained on the Internet by companies such as Medicalogic.

2) Correct Answer B. The HIPAA is intended to standardize medical records so that they can be transferred more easily between doctor's offices, hospitals, insurers etc. Many people, doctors included, feel that this may lead to a significant loss of patient privacy. This is an act mandated by congress.

3) Correct Answer D. Most people sign a waiver when initiating health insurance coverage. This waiver allows access by an employer, the government and auditors at the insurance company. The IRS currently does not have access to your medical records.

4) Correct Answer D. These online health record programs can remind you of important dates, usually by e-mail. These dates might include the due date for your annual physical or dental visit. At this point, you cannot upload any type of graphic data, such as x-rays, although you could keep an x-ray written report online. You can enter and maintain medication information. Finally, you can specify who has access to this information, such as your doctor or family members.

5) Correct answer C. SPAM e-mails which are unsolicited directed e-mail usually contain advertisements. They may also have hyperlinks to send you to a relevant website, when you click. SPAM can, and often does, contain useful information.

SPAM should never contain your credit card information. If it does, it implies that someone has access to this information and that it is being transmitted in an insecure manner around the Internet.

6) Correct Answer D. Registering at a medical website typically entails inputting demographic information such as your email, home address, telephone number, date of birth, etc...This information is used by the medical website for their own promotions and may be sold to an advertiser. When you register, you are usually asked if you would like to receive e-mail from the site, or from one of its advertisers. Simply selecting "No" does not necessarily restrict these e-mails.

7) Correct Answer B. Blood pressure tracking programs allow you to enter your own blood pressure numbers. You can then keep a record of these numbers online. Often, banner advertisements for blood pressure medications are posted on these websites. Specific medications are not recommended. At this point the information is not sent to your doctor, but may be in the future. Although it seems clear that a remote blood pressure device will come into general use in the near future, no such device exists throught the Internet at this time.

8) Corrent answer True, True, True, True, True. Many medical websites use surveys to target advertisements such as banner ads and SPAM. The results may be compiled and posted for general interest. Often, many websites will not allow you to view certain areas or pages until you complete the survey.

9) Correct Answers True, True, True, False, True. Access to your medical information, such as an old EKG can often help you in a life or death situation. You have a right to determine who has access to your medical records, however this right is being eroded by insurance companies and the federal government. Medical records are increasingly being maintained and

transmitted by doctors on the Internet. It is unclear if this transmission is occurring in a private and secure manner. When you move, the doctor can send relevant medical information to your new doctor, if he has access to your chart.

Chapter 5 quiz

1) Which rule is very important in establishing e-mail contact with your doctor?

A) Use e-mail for laboratory value correspondence.

B) Respond to all e-mail from your doctor promptly.

C) Never use e-mail in an emergency situation.

D) Give your doctor an anonymous e-mail address.

2) Uninsured people use the Internet for health information:

A) Less than the insured population.

B) More than the insured population.

C) The same as the insured population.

D) Less than the insured population, but only because they have less access to computers.

3) Which website is not an online physician oriented resource?

A) Medscape.com.

B) Amazon.com.

C) The Doctors Guide to The Internet.

D) Pharminfo.com.

4) Which is not an important legal or ethical issue regarding doctor/physician e-mail?

A) Possible misinformation in e-mail content.

B) Interstate or international boundaries of medical practice.

C) The lack of direct patient contact and examination.

D) All of the above.

5) Which is not a possible advantage for doctors whose patients use the Internet?
   A) potential exposure through patient research to up-to-date medical information.
   B) Lack of control over treatment decisions.
   C) Easier correspondence by e-mail.
   D) Easy access by both doctor and patient to the same resources.

6) Which is a possible indication that your doctor might be resistant to your Internet health research?
   A) He may be dismissive or paternalistic attitude about your findings .
   B) She may ask you to e-mail the information.
   C) He or she relate to you the shortcomings of your particular research.
   D) He or she may tell you that the website you used is unreliable.

7) Evaluative tools to analyze your online health research might include:
   A) A way of determining the credentials of the people presenting the information.
   B) A way to e-mail the information to your doctor.
   C) A method to translate medical terminology.
   D) A method for ensuring the privacy of your research.

8) What types of subjects should never be transmitted by e-mail between you and your doctor?
   A) All subjects can be transmitted.
   B) Sexual information.
   C) Medication history.
   D) Any information that could potentially be read by others.

9) True or False? People turn to the Internet for health information because of:

A) Frustration about the amount of time the doctor spends with you.

B) Frustration about failed treatments.

C) Convenience.

D) Lack of trust in your doctor or health care system.

E) A desire for anonymity, or feelings of embarrassment about a topic.

10) True or False?

A) Physicians are required for their certification to participate in life long education.

B) A doctor licensed in Canada can prescribe a medication in the United States.

C) Once physicians are certified, they are certified for life.

D) Doctors are licensed by country and can practice in any state in the US.

E) A doctor who spends a lot of time with you is better than a doctor who has up-to-date knowledge.

Chapter 5 Answer Key

1) Correct Answer C. E-mail should never be used in an emergency situation. There is too low a likelihood of it being checked on a regular basis. You may use e-mail to relay laboratory values, although confidential measures should be maintained. Although you should use an anonymous e-mail address or a pseudonym for your Internet health research, you do not necessarily have to do this with your doctor.

2) Correct Answer B. Uninsured people are turning to the Internet more than insured people for health care information. This is presumably to substitute for routine medical care. This occurs despite the possibility that the uninsured have less access to computers and the Internet.

3) Correct Answer B. Amazon.com, although selling a lot of medical books, is not a physician oriented resource. The other sites provide a tremendous amount of medical educational information for your doctor.

4) Correct Answer D. The transmission of medical information by e-mail brings up lots of legal and ethical issues beyond privacy. These include malpractice issues, jurisdictional issues and the potential for physicians giving advice and treatment without actually seeing the patient.

5) Correct Answer B. There are many reasons why your doctor may promote your use of the Internet. Amongst these reasons are the potential that you will bring important clinical research information to the doctor. The doctor will be able to correspond with you in an efficient, timely and self-documenting fashion. You both can have access to the same resources and can refer one another to these resources. The doctor may not, however, like losing control over your treatment decisions.

6) Correct Answer A. A quick dismissal of your hard work is a sure sign that a doctor is resistant. Asking that you e-mail the information and in turn reading the information is apropriate. The doctor may critique your research, telling you about its shortcomings or the unreliability. This should not be translated as a rejection of your efforts.

7) Correct Answer A. Evaluative tools can help you better understand and scrutinize the quality of online information. One criterion is determining the credentials of the people presenting the information. These are not tools to e-mail information to your doctor or for translating medical terminology. Although some evaluative tools allow you to scrutinize the privacy of a website, these tools do not ensure this privacy.

8) Correct Answer D. You should not transmit any information that could potentially be read by others. Your email, in addition

to possible Cookie-based analysis, can be read by employers, e-mail server administrators and nurses. There is no substitution for a private conversation with your doctor.

9) Correct Answer: True, True, True, True, True. All of these are reasons for people turning to the Internet

10) Correct Answer True, False, False, False, True. Physicians must participate in "Continuing Medical Information" to remain board certified and for licensure. Doctors cannot prescribe medications across international borders. Doctors must undergo periodic re-certification, except for older doctors who are "grandfathered" into permanent certification. Doctors are licensed by state in the US. A doctor who spends a lot of time with you is doing you no great service if he is not offering you up-to-date medical care.

Chapter 6 Quiz

1) Online resources for comparing hospitals allow you:

A) To compare the treatment success of certain therapies between hospitals.

B) Tell you where to have your surgery.

C) directly measure physician care.

D) Search for on staff physicians at each hospital.

2. Which of the following offenses would not be included in a doctor's disciplinary record:

A) Traffic violations.

B) improper sexual conduct.

C) criminal convictions.

D) substance abuse.

3. Which of the following types of information is not available in doctor-locator web sites?

A) phone numbers.

B) office location.

C) educational training.

D) treatment success.

4.) Ways of evaluating your doctor online include looking up:

A) Customer satisfaction.

B) Disciplinary records.

C) Educational history.

D) All of the above.

5) Physicians' Websites are:

A) Regulated by the American Medical Association.

B) A source for treatment self-referral.

C) restricted from the provision of interstate medical advice.

D) growing steadily.

6) Internet advertising:

A) Is legally binding.

B) Is more expensive than traditional advertising.

C) May be placed on Doctor's websites.

D) Is not used by doctors to promote their practices.

7) Many doctor's websites contain:

A) Links to other online resources.

B) Doctor biographies.

C) Online treatment tools.

D) All of the above.

8) Web site promotion exists through:

A) Referral from other web sites.

B) Search engine registration.

C) Banner advertisement.

D) All of the above.

9) Physician probation is:

A) A period where a doctor's practices are monitored because of a disciplinary issues.

B) A period where a doctor may not practice.

C) Overseen at the federal level.

D) Usually the punishment for repeated disciplinary offenses.

10) True or False?

A) You can obtain information about a physician's board certification at ABMS.org.

B) A physician's board certification is the most important criteria for selecting a doctor.

C) Board certification is automatic for some physicians.

D) Physicians can be certified in more than one specialty.

E) Physicians offering online medical information are certified by a special board.

Chapter 6 Answer Key

1) Correct Answer A. Online hospital comparison websites typically give you information about the success of treatment at a hospital in comparison to nearby hospitals. You can use this information to decide where you might want to have surgery, although you will not be told specifically where to do so. Hospital quality takes more than simply physician care into account when comparing hospitals. Other criteria include nursing care, hospital cleanliness, drug availability, and tertiary services such as x-ray facilities, respiratory care, and physical therapy. Many hospitals maintain their own websites where you can search for staff physicians.

2) Correct Answer A. Traffic violations usually have no bearing on a physician's competency and are not included in online disciplinary records.

3) Correct Answer D. Although there are sites that publish "best doctor" lists, doctor-locator web sites provide general

information such as names, specialties, addresses, and phone numbers, as well as maps to offices, board certifications, medical schools attended, residencies, fellowships, secondary specialties, office hours, languages spoken, affiliated hospitals, and health plans accepted

4) Correct Answer D. Many resources, both objective and subjective are available online to evaluate the quality of your doctor.

5) Correct Answer D. Physician websites are completely unregulated. Theoretically, physicians are restricted from self-referral on their websites just as they are in the rest of their practices. Physicians have been able to render interstate medical advice on their websites. The number of physician websites is rapidly growing because of the low cost and relative ease in setting up a site.

6) Correct Answer A. All advertising, whether it is on the internet or not, is legally binding. Internet based advertising is significantly cheaper than print advertising or TV/radio advertising. Although unregulated at this point, it is theoretically illegal for doctors to place advertisements for any products on their own websites. Doctors are, however promoting their own practices through advertisements on other websites.

7) Correct Answer D. Doctors websites contain many different types of information. At this point, there is no uniformity to doctor websites.

8) Correct Answer D. Each day, new ways of web site promotion are invented. Doctors and hospitals are all taking advantage of these forms of promotion.

9) Correct Answer A. A physician may be placed on probation by his STATE medical board for a first offense. This entails strict monitoring a doctor's practice as he continues to treat

patients. Repeated offenses usually result in suspension or revocation of licensure.

10) Correct Answer True, False, True, True, False. Board Certification information can be obtained online. While board certification implies that a doctor has met criteria set down from a specific medical board, there are many other factors that you should use in selecting a doctor including practice style, bedside manner, education etc. Some doctors have been "grandfathered" in to permanent board certification and do not have to take recertification exams. There is no medical board that oversees online medical information provided by physicians.

Chapter 8 Quiz

1) What types of drugs are restricted on formularies?

A) Cardiac drugs.

B) Cancer chemotherapies.

C) Arthritis medication.

D) All of the above.

2) What resources are available for Internet communication with your health plan?

A) E-mail to claims departments.

B) Online appeals.

C) Explanations of the reasons drugs are placed on formulary.

D) Benefits in comparison to other plans.

3) Which of the following is not a choice for dealing with a claim denial?

A) Specialized litigation.

B) External review.

C) Submitting supporting documentation.

D) Making your doctor pay for it.

4) Although Medicare beneficiaries can see that they are entitled to certain health screening tests:
A) They generally must have a symptom or significant history of a disease before the doctor can obtain the test.
B) They do not need to sign any form of a waiver.
C) They can appeal any denials on-line.
D) They can only have limited tests when they are sick.

5) Step therapy Formularies:
A) Allow you access to any drug.
B) Are not specified on health plan websites.
C) Require you to prove that a formulary drug is not working before advancing to another drug.
D) Allow you to change between formulary drugs at your discretion.

6) Gag clauses for doctors
A) Are still in effect in managed care health plans.
B) Restricted the doctor from discussing the financial arrangement of his contract.
C) Allowed the doctor to discuss all treatment options with the patient.
D) Were abandoned because they were too costly.

7) PPM is:
A) An on-line broker for health insurance.
B) A website for health insurance denials.
C) A business that links insurance and pharmaceutical companies.
D) A measure of drug toxicity.

8) Managed Care treatment service programs:
A) Use the internet to provide information to the patient.
B) Are a resource for the standardization of care.
C) Exist for heart disease and diabetes.

D) All of the above.

9) True or False?

A) Insurance companies are taking the place of many medical websites.

B) Volume discounts are given to insurance companies for purchasing pharmaceuticals.

C) Managed care drug formulary lists are not available on-line.

D) Managed care companies require pre-approval of some medications.

E) Formularies are changed once a year..

10) True or False?

A) Appeals to your insurance company may include documentation from your doctor.

B) You can print out denial claim forms from many websites.

C) Many insurance companies will allow you to check your claim online.

D) Resources are available on the Internet for comparing managed care plans.

E) Many managed care plan websites include information for employers.

Chapter 8 Answer Key

1) Correct Answer D. All types of drugs are restricted on managed care formularies.

2) Correct Answer A. You can often submit an e-mail to the claim department of your health plan. For most plans, this is the only form of on-line communication. Managed care plans do not usually explain why a drug was placed on formulary and do not generally show comparisons to other plans.

3) Correct Answer D. Claim denials should not prompt you to ask your doctor to pay for services or to absorb the cost of

services. There are several avenues available to you following a denial including litigation, external review and gathering and submitting supporting documentation.

4) Correct Answer A. Medicare recipients are only entitled to screening tests—EKGs, PSA, Chest X-rays, etc. when they have an symptom that would prompt the need for the test. It is therefore not a screening test. Medicare recipients must sign a waiver, called an Advanced Beneficiary Waiver Form, which specifies that they will pay for services if the Insurer denies payment for services. Denials of coverage cannot be appealed on line. When a patient is sick with symptoms, Medicare does not generally restrict which tests can be ordered.

5) Correct Answer C. Step therapy formularies are designed so that you try what is usually a less expensive drug for the health plan before using a more expensive one. You thus only have access to some medications. This step therapy plans are clearly outlined on the managed care websites. You can not change drugs at your discretion. Rather, you must wait a mandated amount of time before changing.

6) Correct Answer B. Gag orders have been lifted from almost all managed care plans, allowing a doctor to do what he could not do before-discuss all treatment options with the patient. They were abandoned because of patient and physician resistance.

7) Correct Answer C. PPMs negotiate contracts between insurance and pharmaceutical companies to place drugs on a formulary. PPM is also an abbreviation for parts per million—a measure of environmental toxicity. There are no specific web sites for health insurance denials.

8) Correct Answer D. Managed care treatment service programs are an integrated treatment service provided to customers by each plan. They exist for a variety of long term diseases and allow standardization of care.

9) Correct Answers True, True, False, True, False Most large insurers have their formulary list available on their website. Most managed care companies require pre-approval of some medications. Formalaries may be changed many times a year.

10) Correct Answer True,True,False,True,True

Chapter 9 Quiz

1) What types of drugs are restricted on formularies?

A) Cardiac drugs.

B) Cancer chemotherapies.

C) Arthritis medication.

D) All of the above.

2) What resources are available for Internet communication with your health plan?

A) E-mail to claims departments.

B) Online appeals.

C) Explanation of the reasons drugs are placed on formulary.

D) Benefits in comparison to other plans..

3) Which of the following is not a choice for dealing with a claim denial?

A) Specialized litigation.

B) External review.

C) Submitting supporting documentation.

D) Making your doctor pay for it.

4) Although Medicare beneficiaries can see that they are entitled to certain health screening tests:

A) They must have a symptom or.significant history of a disease before the doctor can obtain the test.

B) They do not need to sign any form of a waiver.

C) They can appeal any denials on-line.

D) They can only have limited tests when they are sick.

5) Step therapy Formularies:

A) Allow you access to any drug.

B) Are not specified on health plan websites.

C) Require you to prove that a formulary drug is not working before advancing to another drug.

D) Allow you to change between formulary drugs at your discretion.

6) Gag clauses for doctors:

A) Are still in effect in managed care health plans.

B) Restricted the doctor from discussing the financial arrangement of his contract.

C) Allowed the doctor to discuss all treatment options with the patient.

D) Were abandoned because they were too costly.

7) A PPM is:

A) An on-line broker for health insurance.

B) A website for health insurance denials.

C) A business that links insurance and pharmaceutical companies.

D) A measure of drug toxicity.

8) Managed Care treatment service programs:

A) Use the internet to provide information to the patient.

B) Are a resource for the standardization of care.

C) Exist for heart disease and diabetes.

D) All of the above.

9) True or False?

A) Insurance companies are taking the place of many medical websites.

B) Volume discounts are given to insurance companies for purchasing pharmaceuticals.

C) Managed care drug formulary lists are not available on-line.

D) Managed care companies require pre-approval of some medications.

E) Formularies are changed once a year.

10) True or False?

A) Appeals to your insurance company may include documentation from your doctor.

B) You can print out denial claim forms from many websites.

C) Many insurance companies will allow you to check your claim online

D) Resources are available on the Internet for comparing managed care plans

E) Many managed care plan websites include information for employers.

Chapter 8 Answer Key

1) Correct Answer D. All types of drugs are restricted on managed care formularies.

2) Correct Answer A. You can often submit an e-mail to the claim department of your health plan. For most plans, this is the only form of on-line communication. Managed care plans do not usually explain why a drug was placed on formulary and do not generally show comparisons to other plans.

3) Correct Answer D. Claim denials should not prompt you to ask your doctor to pay for services or to absorb the cost of services. There are several avenues available to you following a denial including litigation, external review and gathering and submitting supporting documentation.4) Correct Answer A. Medicare recipients are only entitled to screening tests— EKGs, PSA, Chest X-rays, etc. when they have an symptom that would prompt the need for the test. It is therefore not a screening test. Medicare recipients must sign a waiver, called an Advanced Beneficiary Waiver Form, that specifies that they

will pay for services if payment for services is denied by the Insurer. Denials of coverage can not be appealed on line. When a patient is sick with symptoms, Medicare does not generally restrict which tests can be ordered.

5) Correct Answer C. Step therapy formularies are designed so that you try what is usually a less expensive drug for the health plan before using a more expensive one. You thus only have access to some medications. This step therapy plans are clearly outlined on the managed care websites. You can not change drugs at your discretion. Rather, you must wait a mandated amount of time before changing.

6) Correct Answer B. Gag orders have been lifted from almost all managed care plans, allowing a doctor to do what he could not do before—discuss all treatment options with the patient. They were abandoned because of patient and physician resistance.

7) Correct Answer C. PPMs negotiate contracts between insurance and pharmaceutical companies to place drugs on a formulary. PPM is also an abbreviation for parts per million—a measure of environmental toxicity. There are no specific web sites for health insurance denials.

8) Correct Answer D. Managed care treatment service programs are an integrated treatment service provided to customers by each plan. They exist for a variety of long term diseases and allow standardization of care.

9) Correct Answers True, True, False, True, False. Most large insurers have their formulary list available on their website. Most managed care companies require pre-approval of some medications. Formularies may be changed many times a year.

10) Correct Answer True, True, False, True, True

Chapter 9 Quiz

1) Web sites representing offshore pharmacies are:

A) Sites to obtain medication not necessarily approved by the FDA.

B) Regulated by an international commission.

C) Always dispense standardized medications.

D) Not currently accessible from the United States.

2) Telemedicine promises to:

A) Remove the doctor from your medical care.

B) Allow you to watch your doctor performing surgery on television.

C) Link you to your doctor over the Internet or some other electronic medium.

D) Make it more difficult for rural healthcare patients to see their doctor.

3) When obtaining prescriptions for medicine online, you must consider:

A) You can always judge the qualifications of the person making the prescription.

B) Online pharmacies are generally secure private sites.

C) The safety oversight of the FDA, directed by your doctor may be bypassed.

D) That the medication that you order may not be the medication that you receive.

4) The most popular drug prescribed and available on the Internet is:

A) Propecia®—for male pattern baldness.

B) Celebrex®—for arthritis.

C) Xenical®—for weight loss.

D) Viagra®—for erectile dysfunction.

5) Regarding online prescribing:

A) Federal laws exist through the FDA.

B) Many states have vague statutes regarding practicing medicine through electronic means.

C) Prescriptions are made by non-doctors.

D) The patient must send a prescription to the website.

6) Online questionnaires for prescription medications:

A) Are exhaustive and lead you to a diagnosis for which you should see your doctor.

B) Ask important questions to prevent any short-term serious side effects.

C) Ignore other medications which you may be taking.

D) Do not remove liability for the web site.

7) Which of the following is not a form of telemedicine?

A) Having your pacemaker checked through a telephone device.

B) Speaking with your doctor about your symptoms on the telephone.

C) Battlefield surgery using a specialized device by a remote doctor safely behind the frontline.

D) Watching the Discovery Channel®.

8) Which legal issue is not of concern regarding online medical practice?

A) Fraud.

B) Liability.

C) Confidentiality.

D) =Free speech.

9) True or False? Which of the following are potential problems related to Internet based medical care?

A) Examination of the patient.

B) Discussion of treatment alternatives.

C) Establishment of a reliable medical history.

D) Convenience for the patient..

E) Information on risks and benefits.

10) True or False? Which are subtle but important physical exam clues that a doctor uses when seeing the patient?
A) The patient's gait.
B) The patient's mood.
C) The patient's attention span.
D) The patient's willingness to pay for the visit.
E) The patient's fingernails.

Chapter 9 Answer Key

1) Correct Answer A. Offshore pharmacy websites are available to purchase drugs not approved by the US FDA. They are completely unregulated and there is no standardization of the medication dispensed. These websites are accessible from the United States, but are illegal.

2) Correct Answer C. Telemedicine uses tools, whether they be the telephone, internet or some other sophisticated device to link you and your doctor over a distance. It is not intended to remove your doctor from your medical care. Although websites exist for you to observe surgery, Telemedicine is not "televised" medicine. Telemedicine promises to improve the health care for rural healthcare patients by giving them a means of communicating with a doctor over a long distance.

3) Correct Answer C. Although the FDA oversees medications which are sold and dispensed in traditional "brick and mortar" pharmacies, there is no such oversight of online prescriptions. The qualifications of the person making the prescription are not usually easily discerned. These sites are not always secure sights and privacy may be breached. In many instances, patients have described receiving different medications than the one they ordered. It is also possible that you could receive a cheaper substitute for the medication you ordered which is not necessarily equally potent or safe.

4) Correct Answer D. The proliferation of online prescriptions seems to be in medications that patients may be reluctant to ask their physician about. Viagra® is far away the leader in this regard. Also beware, many online prescribers are selling Viagra® substitutes, cleverly worded such as Viagro or "Natural" Viagra

5) Correct Answer B. Many states are just beginning to realize that this form of medication acquisition is completely unregulated. Federal laws do not exist for online prescribing. On many of these websites a paid doctor may oversee your questionnaire. You do not have to send anything to these websites except for your money.

6) Correct Answer B. Online questionnaires at online prescription sites will ask questions about short term side effects and other medication you may be taking. Other than this, they are not exhaustive and generally make it very easy to get a medication prescription. These questionnaires do remove the online prescriber from liability (read the fine print!!)

7) Correct Answer D. Watching medical information on television is not telemedicine. these other forms of medical care are currently being carried out everyday.

8) Correct Answer D. Although free speech is an issue for all Internet based communication, the legal issues specifically related to online medical practice are fraud, liability, confidentiality and licensure.

9) Correct answer True, True, True, False, True. Although telemedicine and online medical care are more convenient for the patient all of the other choices are potential problems associated with this type of care.

10) Correct Answer(s) True, True, True, False, True. There are many important clues that a doctor uses when assessing the health of the patient. These are often subtle and may go

unnoticed by the patient. The patient's unwillingness to pay for the visit is not one of them. An abnormality of the patient's gait may have important implications for a neurological disease. An alternation in the patient's mood may suggest a psychological disturbance. Changes in the patient's fingernails are an excellent clue to long term illness or abrupt onset of disease. Many excellent diagnosticians look at the patient's fingernails as they are shaking their hand in greeting.

Chapter 10 Quiz

1) You must contribute to medication surveillance because:
A) Some of the medications sold online are unsafe.
B) The FDA has brought many medications to market before rigorous pre-market screening.
C) Foreign pharmacies can sell non FDA approved medications.
D) Medication and nutritional product interactions are not significant.

2) Which resource is not available through regulated online pharmacies?
A) An Online medical dictionary.
B) An online prescription reference guide.
C) An online prescription generator.
D) An online medication interaction guide.

3) Online pharmacies work by which of the following mechanisms?
A) Sales of prescription drugs to any state regardless of license.
B) Mail delivery of prescriptions.
C) Submission of a phoned in prescription only.
D) Cheaper prices to consumers.

4) Your consumer habits are important to the online advertisers of drug products because:

a) Having you switch to another drug can be very profitable.

b) Drug companies are all working together.

c) Online advertising fees are the chief form of revenue for online pharmacies.

d) None of the above.

5) Planning ahead when ordering from an online pharmacy is important because:

a) Your doctor expects a delay when starting your medication.

b) Many medication regimens allow for a few days to be skipped in between doses.

c) It may take several days for your medication to be delivered.

d) Your order may take several days to process after the prescription is received.

6) Changes in Medication regimen are likely to affect which type of patients?

A) HIV positive patients.

B) Chronic high blood pressure patients.

C) Patients with under active thyroids.

D) None of the above.

7) Information supplied by online pharmacies is:

A) Allows you to have legal recourse against the pharmacy in case of a side effect.

B) Purely informational.

C) Sometimes helpful in catching a potential mistake by your doctor.

D) The same as you would receive from a traditional pharmacy.

8) Transmitting prescriptions by computer has the potential to eliminate which of the following?

A) pharmacists from dispensing medication.

B) Potential medication errors due to handwriting.

C) Prescription fraud.

D) The need for you to see your doctor.

9) True or False?

A) All online pharmacies should have a registered pharmacist.

B) All online pharmacies will dispense medications without a prescription.

C) All pharmacy websites should have a US address.

D) Some online pharmacies claim that the government is conspiring to supress the sale of a product.

E) Patient testimonies on pharmacy websites are a marker for a reliable source.

10) True or False? People are drawn to online pharmacies because of:

A) Convenience.

B) Cost.

C) Availability of medications.

D) Privacy.

E) The ability to purchase non-medication items.

Chapter 10 Answer Key

Correct Answer D. There are many important and potentially unsafe interactions between medications and nutritional products. Many online pharmacies sell non-FDA approved and sometimes unsafe medications. Many medications have been approved by the FDA and subsequently removed from the market because of post-release problems.

2) Correct Answer C. Prescriptions should only come from your doctor. Many online pharmacies have excellent online resources for researching medication.

3) correct Answer B. Prescriptions are always mailed, either in the regular mail, by parcel or by express mail. Online pharmacies

can only send prescriptions from their home state to states where they maintain an out-of-state license. Doctors can submit phoned in prescriptions or send them by computer. Customers must submit written proof of their prescription, either by fax or mail. Despite claims to the contrary, most online pharmacies are not cheaper than traditional pharmacies, except for some selected medication.

4) Correct Answer A. If you ask your doctor to switch you from one drug to another, this can be very profitable for one drug company and very costly for another. Drug companies are in intense competition with one another. Most of the online pharmacies generate their revenue chiefly from sales, not from ad fees.

5) Correct Answer C. Ordering from an online pharmacy requires you to transmit you prescription either by mail or by fax. Your doctor usually expects you to start your medication immediately. Almost all medications need to be taken at least on a daily basis, and no doses should be skipped. Because your medication is mailed, it may take several days for your medication to be delivered.

6) Correct answer A. HIV therapy changes frequently. As this disease is increasingly being viewed as a treatable, survivable disease, it is imperative that patients be taking the correct medications. Many. Although new blood pressure medications are constantly released, many high blood pressure patients have been stably taking the same medication for many years and should probably not be changed. The same reasoning applies for the treatment of hypothyroidism.

7) Correct Answer B. Information provided by online pharmacies is purely informational. You are often required to sign a waiver of liability before viewing certain information. There is a tremendous amount of information that can be received from an online pharmacy information. This is usually a lot more

than what is available from traditional pharmacies. Sometimes this information can serve to supplement the information that your receive from your doctor and sometimes it can alert you to a mistake by your doctor (i.e. a medication interaction)

8) Correct Answer B. Transmitting prescriptions by computer may eliminate the errors of a doctor's poor handwriting. Many prescription mistakes are made each year because of this problem. Pharmacists will still need to dispense the medication and you will usually still need to see your doctor before receiving a prescription. No one knows how easy it may be to transmit false prescriptions.

9) Correct Answer True, False, True, True, False You should confirm that an online pharmacy has an registered pharmacist on staff before purchasing medication. Although there are several online pharmacies that will dispense medication without a prescription, the majority will not do so. If you are purchasing medication as a US resident, you need, according to federal law, purchase from a pharmacy within the US. Some online pharmacies promote products with ridiculous claims about suppressed products by the government and industry. Patient testimonies should be avoided as unreliable and difficult to confirm.

10) Correct Answer True, True, True, True, True. There are many reasons that online pharmacies have grown so rapidly in popularity. All of these answers are supported by consumer opinion.

Appendix B—Assignments

Chapter 1
Go to some of the large Medical Websites and Surf around these sites. Do so without registering. We will discuss registering in a latter Chapter. Check out WebMD.com, HealthCentral.com, DrKoop.com and Dicoveryhealth.com.

Chapter 2
Perform a search on different databases using the search terms. Try entering the terms "smoking" and "lung disease" in several different search engines. Try this in Yahoo.com, Altavista.com,. WebMD.com, and NIH.gov. Try to determine why the results are so different.

Chapter 3
Find your cookie folder and empty it. Within days of surfing, however, it will be refilled. You should also attempt to set the security profiles on your browser through the Options menu.

Chapter 4
Try to identify SPAM in your e-mail folder. See if you can figure out what they are trying to sell and where it came from. Try to remember if this SPAM was initiated by a website where you may have visited.

Chapter 5
Ask your doctor about any standardized methods he or she may have to communicate with you via the Internet. Write a letter to

your doctor to suggest ways that patient—generated Internet health research may be used in a constructive streamlined manner.

Chapter 6

Compare the local hospitals in your area by using a web resource such as Healthgrades.com.

Chapter 7

If you are part of a large health plan, find their website. Usually it is simply the name of the plan followed by .com. Once you are on the site, look for the drug formulary and an explanation of your benefits.

Chapter 8

If you are part of a large health plan, find their website. Usually it is simply the name of the plan followed by .com. Once you are on the site, look for the drug formulary and an explanation of your benefits.

Chapter 9

Go to an online prescribing site and read the liability statements and disclaimers.

Chapter 10

Look up the medications you are taking on a pharmacy website. Do a cost comparison between sites and to the way you are currently receiving medication

www.ingramcontent.com/pod-product-compliance
Lightning Source LLC
Chambersburg PA
CBHW061246280526
45784CB00002B/657